Dr Penny Stanway practised for several years as a GP and as a child-health doctor before becoming increasingly fascinated by researching and writing about a healthy diet and other natural approaches to health and wellbeing. She is an accomplished cook who very much enjoys being creative in the kitchen and sharing food with others. Penny has written more than 20 books on health, food and the connections between the two. She lives with her husband in a houseboat on the Thames and often visits the south-west of Ireland. Her leisure pursuits include painting, swimming and being with her family and friends.

By the same author:

The Miracle of Cider Vinegar
The Miracle of Lemons
The Miracle of Bicarbonate of Soda
The Natural Guide to Women's Health
Healing Foods for Common Ailments
Good Food for Kids
Free Your Inner Artist

As co-author:
Breast is Best
Christmas – A Cook's Tour
The Lunchbox Book

THE MIRACLE OF
OLIVE OIL

Practical Tips for
HEALTH, HOME
& BEAUTY

DR PENNY STANWAY

WATKINS PUBLISHING
LONDON

This edition first published in the UK and USA 2012 by
Watkins Publishing, Sixth Floor, Castle House,
75–76 Wells Street, London W1T 3QH

1 3 5 7 9 10 8 6 4 2

Designed and typeset by Jerry Goldie Graphic Design

Printed and bound by Imago in China

British Library Cataloguing-in-Publication Data Available

Library of Congress Cataloging-in-Publication Data Available

ISBN: 978-1-78028-105-6

www.watkinspublishing.co.uk

Distributed in the USA and Canada by Sterling Publishing Co., Inc.
387 Park Avenue South, New York, NY 10016-8810

For information about custom editions, special sales, premium and
corporate purchases, please contact Sterling Special Sales
Department at 800-805-5489 or specialsales@sterlingpub.com

Contents

This book is dedicated to every cook whose effort and thoughtfulness make the most of the oils, vinegars, fruits, vegetables, meat, fish, grains, sugars and spices that we are so blessed to have.

Acknowledgements

Thank you to my sister, Jenny Hare, for her joy in food and cooking; to my husband, Andrew, for his unstinting enthusiasm in discussing olive oil; to my family and friends for their good company and warm-heartedness when sharing the food I've cooked; to my agent, Doreen Montgomery, for her endless encouragement and support; and to my editor, Alison Bolus, for her patience, wisdom and good sound common sense.

Introduction

Is olive oil truly a miracle, you may ask? Well, arguably it is – if we define a miracle as an amazing or wonderful occurrence.

Olive oil's colour is attractive, its smell is delightful, its flavour is luscious and unusual, its feel in the mouth and on the skin is sensual and its light (from an olive-oil lamp) is soft and glowing. In addition, olive oil (as part of a healthy diet) can help to prevent and treat many ailments, thanks to constituents such as its monounsaturated fats and antioxidant polyphenols.

In this book there is much to discover about olive oil, including where it comes from, what is in it, its health benefits, and its use as a beauty aid and in cooking. Finally, there are lots of recipes, all of them containing olive oil as an important ingredient.

So valuable a commodity has olive oil been over the centuries that it is easy to understand why Homer called olive oil 'liquid gold' in the 'Odyssey', and why the 'father' of medicine, Hippocrates, referred to it as 'the great healer'.

CHAPTER 1

Olive oil

This hugely popular oil comes from the fruits of the olive tree, which is known to botanists as *Olea europaea* – '*olea*' being Latin for 'oil'. The fruits are olives, and both their pulp and their stones are oily; indeed, oil forms 12–30 per cent of the fruit pulp and 10–12 per cent of the stone, depending on the ripeness and variety. Besides being oily, olives are also bitter, thanks mainly to a substance called oleuropein. Some of this is present in olive oil, making this slightly bitter too.

Olive oil is highly prized as a food, a source of light (when burned in a lamp), a medicine and a beauty aid. For millennia it has been carried up and down the trading routes of Asia and Europe. Christopher Columbus took olive oil to America in 1492, and today it is exported from olive-growing countries to consumers around the world, with its markets growing year by year. However, consumers are also becoming more sophisticated in their choice of olive oil and are seeking higher grades that have more flavour as well as a higher content of polyphenols and other health-giving substances.

History

Experts have dated fossilized olive leaves found on certain Greek islands to an astonishing 50–60,000 years old! Many believe that wild olive trees first grew in what is now eastern Turkey, though others think they originated in North Africa. Olive trees were eventually cultivated in order to improve their yield.

Phoenician, Roman and Arabic traders took olive trees to nearby countries, known today as Algeria, France, Greece, Iran, Iraq, Israel, Italy, Lebanon, Libya, Morocco, Pakistan, Portugal, Saudi Arabia, Spain, Syria and Tunisia. Spanish and Portuguese explorers exported olive trees to the West Indies in the 15th and 16th centuries and later to the Americas. In the late 18th century, Franciscan missionaries introduced them to California. Today, olive trees are also grown in Australia, China, Japan and South Africa, but the country that produces more olive oil than anywhere else is Spain, with Greece and Italy tying in second place.

Geography

Olive trees require hot dry summers, mild wet winters, well-drained soil, enough wind for pollination, and irrigation during the growing season. All these conditions are found in Mediterranean countries and at equivalent distances from the Equator in the Americas, Africa and Australia.

Symbolism

The olive tree, or often just an olive branch (as in 'offering an olive branch'), is sometimes used as a symbol of peace. The tree is also a symbol of wisdom. Picasso's image of a dove carries a sprig from an olive tree. The olive is a sign of peace, friendship, wisdom, glory, power, fertility and purity. Kings and queens are annointed with olive oil to symbolize their authority. And two other names for Jesus – the 'Messiah' and the 'Christ' – mean 'one annointed with olive oil' in Hebrew and Greek, respectively.

Olive oil in the last 50 years

Around 50 years ago, scientists linked the traditional diet in southern Italy and Crete with a reduced risk of heart disease. Since then, others have associated this with a reduced risk of many other health conditions. This diet is dubbed the 'Mediterranean Diet', and olive oil is one of several of its components that aid health. Indeed, Cretans consume a very large amount of olive oil, with figures from 1996 revealing that the average Cretan adult consumed 31 litres (more than 54 pints) a year.

Other studies (see Chapter 4) suggest that olive oil on its own can also aid good health.

During the last 50 years there has been exponential interest around the world in using fresh, well-produced culinary ingredients, such as extra virgin olive oil. And just as some people delight in getting to know and enjoy different wines, so, too, are increasing numbers of people now fascinated by tasting and using different olive oils.

CHAPTER 2

Growing and pressing olives

Thousands of people around the world grow olive trees so that they can enjoy their fruits and their oil. Many have only a few trees and produce olives and oil for just their personal use, whilst others farm much larger numbers of olive trees in order to sell their produce. Some farms have their own olive presses, but other growers send their olives to local communal presses or to larger, more industrialized olive treatment centres.

Growing olive trees

Olive farmers choose their variety of olive according to the size and flavour of the olives they want to produce. They need the right climate and soil to grow their crop successfully. Finally, a water supply is important, too, as rainfall isn't always sufficient.

Another important factor is how to control pests such as insects and fungi, which can damage the trees, their leaves or the olives. However, rather than use fertilizers and commercial pesticides, with their risk for both labourers and consumers, growers are increasingly turning to organic farming methods.

Olive trees need to be about 15–20 years old before they yield worthwhile crops of olives, but they then continue producing well – usually with a good crop every other year – until they are about 80 years old or even, it is believed, up to 500 years! In fact, they may live for hundreds if not thousands of years, since new growth continually sprouts from the base of the trunk.

About 90 per cent of the world's olives are used to make olive oil.

Harvesting the olives

At harvest time, labourers spread nets or plastic tarpaulins on the ground, then either hand-pick the olives (which is, inevitably, expensive) or encourage ripe olives to fall by raking or beating the trees, or using an electric branch comb. They may even use a mechanical tree or branch shaker attached to a catching frame. The more carefully the olives are harvested, the better the quality of the oil. This is because rough handling makes olive oil more acidic by encouraging its fats to break down and release free fatty acids.

As they ripen, olives change colour from green to purple to black (or from green to red). Olives picked before they are fully ripe tend to produce oil that is green, while ripe olives produce a yellower, sweeter oil. Also, less-ripe olives produce smaller amounts of oil than do ripe ones. The olives are transported to a processing plant as soon as possible. This is partly because any delay encourages fermentation, which increases the acidity of the olives, and partly because it encourages the breakdown of antioxidants such as vitamin E and polyphenols in the oil.

The olives are then washed to get rid of dirt, leaves and twigs.

Pressing the olives

In olden times, olives were crushed by a round millstone turned by donkeys (or, in certain countries, by slaves), and the oil was squeezed from the crushed olives by a screw press. Three separate pressings were needed to remove all the oil. The first pressing produced the best oil, known as *extra virgin oil*. The second and third pressings produced slightly less good oil, both called *virgin oil*. (In some areas, producers mixed hot water into the olive paste remaining after the first and second pressings to make it easier to extract the oil.)

Some small-scale processing plants still produce olive oil in a similar way, though the millstones have been replaced by a mashing hammer and the screw press by a hydraulic press that extracts oil in one pressing.

Oil produced in these ways is called 'cold-pressed' as long as the temperature of the olive paste has never exceeded 28°C (82°F). Such oil is generally allowed to age for three weeks in the dark before being offered for consumption and has a shelf life of two to three years.

However, many modern processing plants do things differently. They crush the olives in an electric crusher, then choose one of three methods to extract the oil: mill the paste to squeeze out the oil, centrifuge the paste to spin out the oil, or use a machine that attracts oil molecules by surface tension. Some processing plants add water to the crushed olives. Unfortunately, antioxidant polyphenols from the olives' oil dissolve into the water and the antioxidant-laden water is eventually discarded, leaving the oil depleted of these health-promoting and flavour-enhancing constituents. This also results in a shorter shelf life, because the antioxidant polyphenols would have delayed rancidity.

The oil that runs from the mill first is best because it has an excellent flavour, the lowest acidity and the highest antioxidant levels. Its quality is equivalent to that of the extra virgin oil produced by the first pressing of a screw press. So, to maintain tradition, it is called *extra virgin oil.*

The oil produced later in the milling process is of a very high quality, with a good flavour, but with slightly more acidity and slightly lower antioxidant levels. Its quality is equivalent to that of the virgin oil traditionally produced by the second and third pressings of a screw press, and to maintain tradition it is called *virgin oil.*

The oil that emerges from the mill is still mixed with the water that was used to soften the crushed olives, and this water must be removed. One method is to decant the oil as it rises to the surface of the oil/water mixture. Another is to spin the mixture in an electric centrifuge.

Olive pomace oil, which is the lowest grade of all the olive oils, differs from extra virgin olive oil, virgin olive oil, ordinary virgin olive oil (see below), refined olive oil, and olive oil. It is produced by means of a solvent such as hexane, which extracts the oil from the pomace.

Filtering

Olive oil is sometimes filtered to remove the cloudiness that results from suspended particles of olive pulp – or the sludge that would be formed by such particles sinking to the bottom of a container of oil. Some people think that unfiltered oil tastes better; others say it makes no difference. However, filtered oil keeps its flavour longer and deteriorates less quickly.

Refining

Poorer-quality olive oils can be refined to reduce their acidity and any unpleasant flavour or high colour. This can be done with caustic soda (sodium hydroxide) but is increasingly being done by physical methods such as centrifuging ('spinning') it and/or heating it in a vacuum to 180°C (350°F).

Grades of olive oil and olive pomace oil

In 2010, the United States Department of Agriculture released new regulations on the grading and labelling of olive oil and olive pomace oil. These are largely based on those from the International Olive Council (IOC) in Madrid – which in turn are recognized by the vast majority of the world's olive-oil producers and marketers. The IOC regulations differentiate olive oils into four grades and several sub-grades, each with specific requirements as to their production method, colour, odour, flavour, peroxide value (indicating the amount of oxidation) and acidity (measured as its content of free oleic acid), moisture, impurities and trace metals.

Virgin olive oils

These are obtained by pressing or other physical means, under conditions that do not alter the oil, from olives that have undergone no treatment other than washing, decanting, centrifuging and filtering. The less acidic the oil and the higher the number of phenols, the better its quality.

- *Extra virgin olive oil* has a maximum free acidity of 0.8g per 100g, and contains 366mg of phenols per kg.

- *Virgin olive oil* has a maximum free acidity of 2g per 100g, and contains 164mg of phenols per kg.

- *Ordinary virgin olive oil* has a maximum free acidity of 3.3g per 100g.

- *Lampante olive oil* is used in industry; it is edible only if refined (see below); its free acidity is more than 3.3g per 100g.

Refined olive oils

These are obtained by refining lampante olive oil to remove its free fatty acids (and therefore its acidity) without altering its fats. One method is to centrifuge it, then heat it in a vacuum to evaporate away its fatty acids. Refined olive oils have a maximum free acidity of 0.3g per 100g, and contain only 2.7mg of phenols per kg.

'Olive oil'

This is a blend of refined olive oil and virgin olive oil (though not lampante); its maximum free acidity is 1g per 100g. Its name, which is specific to this blend, is easily confused with the generic term 'olive oil' and it is a pity that the new regulations did not address this.

Olive pomace oil

This is usually obtained by treating olive pomace with a solvent such as trichlorothylene:

- Crude olive pomace oil is edible only if refined.

- Refined olive pomace oil is obtained by refining crude pomace oil to remove its acidity without altering its fats (for example, by centrifuging then heating); its maximum free acidity is 0.3g per 100g.

- Olive pomace oil is a blend of refined olive pomace oil and virgin olive oil (not lampante); its maximum free acidity is 1g per 100g.

Refined olive oils have no odour or flavour, and 'olive oils' and olive pomace oils have little or none.

Other processing

Old or rancid olive oils, or oils from diseased or otherwise poor-quality olives, can be made palatable by filtering, heating, or treating with charcoal or chemicals to adjust their acidity.

Stones or no stones?

Most olive oil is made from olives that are crushed together with their stones. Some, though, is made from stoned olives. Both types have advocates who claim that their preferred oil tastes better or lasts longer.

Labelling

There is increasing interest in where the olives that contributed to a bottle of olive oil were grown and pressed. A decree in Italy in 2007 stated that every bottle of Italian oil must declare where the olives came from, where they were pressed, and the presence of any additional vegetable oils. However, in February 2008, European Union officials ruled that such labelling need only be voluntary. 'Single-estate' oils are generally more expensive than oils made from pooled sources.

Scandals

Over the years, there have been several scandals when olive oils have been discovered to have been adulterated with a lower-grade olive oil than indicated on the label, or with other vegetable oils.

An article in *The New Yorker* (13 August 2007) by journalist Tom Mueller alleged that regulation in Italy was extremely lax, major Italian shippers regularly adulterated olive oil, only about 40 per cent of the oil sold as 'extra virgin olive oil' met the specification, and colza (Swedish turnip – or swede) oil containing added colour and flavour had sometimes been passed off as olive oil. Since then, the Italian police have been particularly vigilant. For example, seven olive-oil processing plants were impounded and 40 people arrested in Italy in 2008 for adding chlorophyll to sunflower and soya bean oil and passing it off as extra virgin olive oil.

CHAPTER 3

What's in olive oil

The vast bulk of olive oil – 99.9 per cent, in fact – is formed of fats, which are also known as triglycerides (or triacylglycerols). Each tablespoon (15ml) of the oil contains 119 calories of energy, virtually all from fat. Besides being the main constituent of olive oil, fat is also the main nutrient in the oil, the others including certain vitamins and traces of certain minerals. Olive oil also contains free fatty acids that have come from the breakdown of some of its fats, as well as fatty substances called phospholipids, glycerol (glycerine) and waxes.

Other constituents include polyphenols, flavonoids, pigments, terpenes, organic acids, sterols and flavour compounds, many of which are antioxidants. The amounts of these constituents of olive oil are mostly low compared with those in vegetables and fruits, but are none-theless useful. They are highest in unrefined olive oils (extra virgin and virgin olive oils) and much lower in refined olive oils, other seed and vegetable oils, margarine, 'spreads', butter and lard.

Minute fragments of olives contribute to the cloudiness of many extra virgin olive oils.

Olive oil may also contain unwanted substances such as peroxides and polycyclic aromatic hydrocarbons, especially if it has been badly treated.

The exact composition of olive oil varies according to the type of olive and the soil, altitude, climate, ripeness of the olives, time-lag and care between olive picking and oil extraction, and method of extraction.

The chemistry of fats

Each molecule of fat in olive oil comprises one glycerol molecule and three fatty-acid molecules. The fatty acids are either *saturated*, meaning their atoms are connected by single electro-chemical bonds, or *unsaturated*, meaning they contain one or more double bonds. A *monounsaturated* fatty acid contains one double bond, a *polyunsaturated* fatty acid more than one. Double bonds enable fatty acid molecules to bend, making them vitally important components of cell membranes. But double bonds also make molecules less stable, so more prone to oxidation by light, heat, air or particular biochemical factors in the body. The number in the names of the three groups of unsaturated fatty acids – omega-3 and omega-6 polyunsaturated fatty acids, and omega-9 monounsaturated fatty acids – denotes the position of the first double bond in the molecule.

The fats we eat

Experts say that our diet should contain a certain proportion of fat and a good balance of fatty acids in that fat. They generally agree that the average westernized diet contains too much fat in total, of which too much is polyunsaturated fat and not enough is monounsaturated fat. Many, though not all (see pages 14 and 21), believe that too much saturated fat is a problem.

For example:

- The Department of Agriculture in the US recommends that an adult's fat intake provides 20–35 per cent of their calories. Less than 10 per cent of calories should come from saturated fats; and most fats should come from polyunsaturated and monounsaturated fats in sources such as fish, nuts and culinary oils.

- The Department of Health in the UK recommends that an adult's fat intake provides no more than 35 per cent of their calories. Less than 11 per cent of calories should be from saturated fat.

(Young children need a higher proportion of fat; so, for example, fat should provide 40 per cent of the calorie intake of the average child under three years old.)

Other experts assert that consuming too much fat, saturated fat in particular, is not the problem. Instead, they say that many people don't consume enough fat that is rich in monounsaturated fatty acids and omega-3 polyunsaturated fatty acids. They also stress that many of us consume too much trans fat.

Trans fat

Also called *hydrogenated* or *partially hydrogenated* fat, trans fat contains polyunsaturated fatty acids that have been heated to very high temperatures to alter their structure and make them hard. Food manufacturers use trans fat to make margarines and spreads and to improve the shelf life of various foods. The danger is that they encourage atherosclerosis (see 'Heart attacks' and 'Strokes' in Chapter 4). They are most often found in fast foods, margarine, vegetable shortening and commercially baked goods. Thankfully, many countries, including the UK, now insist on food labels noting their presence, so consumers can opt not to buy foods containing them. Also, food manufacturers increasingly avoid using them.

'Essential' fatty acids

These are so called because the body cannot make them, so we must get them from our diet.

There are two groups:

- Omega-6s – the main one being linoleic acid

- Omega-3s – the main one being alpha-linolenic acid

Oxidation in our body of omega-6 and omega-3 fatty acids produces omega-6 and omega-3 eicosanoids called prostaglandins, prostacyclins, leukotrienes and thromboxanes. These are known as *signalling molecules*. They help to control inflammation, immunity, body temperature, hormone production and nerve-message transmission. Omega-6 eicosanoids mostly encourage inflammation, while omega-3 eicosanoids are much less inflammatory. Importantly, the balance of omega-6 and omega-3 eicosanoids helps determine whether we get diseases such as arthritis, high blood pressure and cardiovascular disease.

Our balance of omega-6 and omega-3 eicosanoids depends on the balance of omega-6s and omega-3s in our food. Scientists recommend that we eat two to four times as much omega-6 as omega-3. However, the typical western diet provides 10 to 20 (or more) times as much omega-6 as omega-3. So the average omega-6 intake is much too high for optimal health.

Why are the fats in olive oil good for us?

Experts agree that the average diet can be improved by consuming olive oil in place of other culinary oils, hard margarine and spreads. There are three reasons. First, olive oil is high in monounsaturated and low in polyunsaturated fatty acids; second, it contains a better balance of omega-6 and omega-3 fatty acids than most other oils; and third, it has no trans fatty acids.

Olive oil's fats are high in monounsaturated and low in polyunsaturated fatty acids

This means there is less oxidation of the body's fatty acids; a better fatty-acid balance in cholesterol and therefore less risk of it being oxidized; and a better balance of the two main sorts of particle (HDL-cholesterol and LDL-cholesterol) that carry cholesterol in the blood.

Olive oil's fatty acids oxidize less than do those of most other oils

Olive oil's high content of monounsaturated fatty acids and low content of polyunsaturated fatty acids makes it much less prone than most other oils to oxidation, a chemical process that spoils oil by altering its structure. This is because most other oils have a higher proportion of polyunsaturated fatty acids, and these oxidize more quickly than monounsaturated fatty acids.

Oxidation outside the body makes oil rancid. Oxidation inside the body occurs continually in our cells and fluids. Normally, antioxidants (such as vitamin E) restrain it enough to prevent an oxidation-induced cascade of biochemical events, leading to inflammation. However, smoking, stress and a poor diet encourage excessive oxidation. The resulting inflammation encourages many problems, including cardio-vascular disease (see 'Heart disease', page 49, and 'Strokes', page 72), nerve damage and, perhaps, certain cancers.

Olive oil encourages a better balance of fatty acids in cholesterol, and therefore less risk of cholesterol being oxidized

Cholesterol is vital for the production of vitamin D, steroid hormones, neurotransmitters (nerve-message carriers) and bile acids. It helps to create and maintain strong, flexible cell membranes that enable the optimal passage of nutrients, hormones and waste products, and good communication between cells. It's an important part of the myelin sheath, which is vital to the action of many nerves. Finally, it is needed for the production of coenzyme Q10, a vitamin-like substance necessary for energy production.

For optimal health, we need a good balance of the two main types of carrier-particle that transport cholesterol in the blood. Cholesterol and fatty acids are insoluble in water, so to travel safely in the blood they are encased by protein to form particles of either low-density lipoprotein cholesterol (LDL-cholesterol) or high-density lipoprotein cholesterol (HDL-cholesterol). LDL-cholesterol takes cholesterol around the body to the cells. HDL-cholesterol takes excess cholesterol from the cells to the liver, which excretes it in bile. Both LDL- and HDL-cholesterol are therefore vitally important.

Any one person's HDL-cholesterol and LDL-cholesterol carry the same proportions of fatty acids, and these fatty acids are present in the same proportions as in their diet. So because monounsaturated fatty acids are less prone than polyunsaturated ones to oxidation, a person who consumes a higher proportion of monounsaturated fatty acids has some protection against inflammation and related diseases.

GRAMS OF FATTY ACIDS IN 1 TABLESPOON OF OIL OR FAT

	Monounsaturated	Polyunsaturated	Saturated
Olive oil	10.0	1.2	1.8
Rapeseed (canola) oil	8.2	4.1	0.9
Peanut (ground nut) oil	6.2	4.3	2.3
Lard (pork fat)	5.8	1.4	5.0
Chicken fat	5.7	2.6	3.8
Beef fat	5.4	0.5	6.4
Sesame oil	5.4	5.6	1.9
Margarine (tub)	5.2	3.8	2.0
Palm oil	4.4	1.2	5.7
Margarine (block)	4.2	2.4	1.6
Corn (maize) oil	3.3	8.0	1.7
Butter	3.3	0.5	7.2
Soyabean oil	2.9	9.0	0.7
Sunflower oil	2.7	8.9	1.4
Walnut oil	2.6	9.4	8.0
Cottonseed oil	2.5	7.7	3.8
Safflower oil	1.4	10.9	1.7
Coconut oil	0.8	0.2	11.8

Olive oil encourages a better balance of HDL- and LDL-cholesterol

Different fatty acids have different effects on our HDL- and LDL-cholesterol levels (which together add up to give our total cholesterol level) and on our ratio of total cholesterol to HDL-cholesterol. Our goal should be to keep this 'cholesterol ratio' at 5:1 or below, the ideal being below 3.5:1. A healthy ratio discourages atherosclerosis.

Olive oil's high content of monounsaturated fatty acids and low contents of polyunsaturated and saturated fatty acids make it by far the best culinary oil or fat in terms of encouraging a healthy cholesterol ratio.

Some people dub LDL-cholesterol 'bad' cholesterol. However, it's a danger only if:

- It is oxidized. If a person's main dietary fat is olive oil, a high proportion of the fatty acids in their LDL-cholesterol is mono-unsaturated. This is good because monounsaturated fatty acids are much less prone to oxidation than polyunsaturated ones.

- There is too much of it compared with the amount of HDL-cholesterol. This is because HDL-cholesterol removes excess cholesterol by transporting it to the liver, whereas LDL-cholesterol does not.

Most doctors believe that a high total cholesterol is bad and a low one is good, making this the 'official' position. But several studies now suggest that a low total cholesterol is a threat to life, so it is being questioned by more and more experts.

In 2009, *Clinical Cardiology* reported on a US study of 84,429 people, which associated a high total cholesterol level with a lower risk of dying while hospitalized with a heart attack or 'unstable' angina (heart pain). Earlier, in 2004, an Austrian study by the *Journal of Women's Health* of 149,650 people aged 20–95 associated a very low cholesterol level with an increased risk of dying from cancer, liver disease or psychiatric disease, in men of all ages and in women over 50.

Olive oil has a better balance of omega-6 and omega-3 fatty acids than do most other oils

The amounts of omega-6s and omega-3s in olive oil – as in most other common culinary oils – are relatively small, and the ratio of omega-6s to omega-3s is overbalanced towards omega-6. However, the omega-3s can nonetheless be useful, and the ratio is more favourable than that of many other common oils – including corn and sunflower.

The fatty acids most likely to be in short supply in the average diet are the omega-3s. So check that you consume some rich sources, such as oily fish; beef, milk and cheese from grass-fed cows; eggs from free-range hens; leafy green vegetables; walnuts; and linseed (flaxseed).

THE EFFECT OF DIETARY FATTY ACIDS ON HDL-, LDL- AND TOTAL CHOLESTEROL LEVELS AND THE TOTAL HDL RATIO

Fatty acid	HDL-c level	LDL-c level	Total c level	Total: HDL ratio
Monounsaturated	same	down or up	down	much improved
Polyunsaturated	down	down	down	no change
Saturated	up	up	up	no change
Trans	down	may go up	may go up	worse

RATIO OF OMEGA-6 TO OMEGA-3 FATTY ACIDS IN SOME COMMON OILS AND FATS

Butter from grass-fed cows	1.5:1
Mutton fat	1.7:1
Rapeseed (canola) oil	2:1
Soyabean oil	7:1
Lard	7:1
Butter – ordinary	8:1
Beef tallow	8:1
Olive oil	10:1
Walnut oil	15:1
Chicken fat	15:1
Peanut oil	26:1
Corn oil	61:1
Sesame oil	84:1
Cottonseed oil	120:1
Sunflower oil	extremely high, as almost no omega-3s
Safflower oil	extremely high, as almost no omega-3s
Coconut oil	extremely high, as almost no omega-3s
Palm oil	extremely high, as almost no omega-3s

Olive oil has no trans fatty acids

Unlike some margarines and spreads, olive oil contains no trans fat. Some experts would argue that another reason why olive oil can aid health is because it has a very low saturated-fat content compared with that of margarines, spreads, butter and lard. Others, however, believe this is unimportant, pointing to research that suggests that saturated fats are not of themselves the danger to health they were once believed to be.

In summary, we can encourage healthy cholesterol levels and good health in general by consuming olive oil instead of sunflower, corn, rapeseed and other oils containing relatively low levels of mono-unsaturated fatty acids and relatively high levels of polyunsaturated fatty acids.

Free fatty acids, glycerine and waxes

Olive oil is slightly acidic. This acidity is largely caused by free fatty acids released by air, light or heat breaking down triglycerides into free fatty acids and glycerol.

Significant acidity is most common when olives are:

- infested with fruit flies

- infected with fungi

- damaged

- left too long between harvesting and pressing (sometimes on purpose to encourage enzymatic breakdown of the olives and so facilitate oil release)

or when their oil is:

- carelessly extracted

- not removed quickly enough from the watery 'broth' during processing.

Olive oil's acidity clearly reflects the care taken by the olive farmer and the oil producer. The more acidic it is, the more chemical degradation there has been. The acidity of oil from sound, healthy, freshly picked olives, pressed carefully and without delay or heat, is normally very low, at under 0.5 per cent.

Since olive oil, like other vegetable oils, is insoluble in water, its acidity can't be measured in terms of pH (hydrogen ion concentration. Instead, its acidity is measured as the percentage of free fatty acids (the main one being oleic acid) in the oil. An olive oil with a lower percentage of free fatty acids is less acidic than an olive oil with a higher percentage.

Olive oil also contains small amounts of glycerine and waxes.

Antioxidants

These help to prevent oxidation of the fatty acids in olive oil. In addition, they (or their breakdown products, after they have been digested) help to prevent oxidation of the fatty acids in our body. The antioxidants in extra virgin olive oil include polyphenols (see page 25), including oleocanthal and oleuropein (see 'Scent and flavour compounds', page 29), vitamin E (see 'Vitamins', below), flavonoids such as quercetin (see page 27), squalene (see 'Terpenes and terpenoids', page 28) and the plant pigment chlorophyll (see pages 27–8).

Fatty acids can be oxidized by:

- Auto-oxidation – oxidation in the absence of air, caused by electro-chemical reactions creating free radicals (also known as 'reactive oxygen species'). Olive oil's antioxidants prevent this temporarily, but their levels eventually fall. This allows more rapid oxidation, which soon makes the oil rancid.

- Photo-oxidation – oxidation in oil exposed to light. This happens up to 30,000 times faster than auto-oxidation.

Anti-inflammatory compounds

The anti-inflammatory constituents of olive oil include antioxidants and monounsaturated fats. The latter decrease our body's production of inflammatory compounds (such as eicosanoids and cytokines), whereas omega-6 polyunsaturated fats, saturated fats and trans fats do the opposite.

Vitamins

Olive oil contains the fat-soluble vitamins D, E (as tocopherols) and K, plus fat-soluble pro-vitamins called beta carotenes, which are plant pigments that the body converts into vitamin A. Vitamin C and other water-soluble vitamins in olives are almost entirely removed when olives are processed to produce oil.

Olive oil is a good source of vitamin E, with 1 tablespoon containing 1–2mg, which is 10–20 per cent of the recommended daily intake. Vitamin E can be stored for long periods in our body fat and our liver.

Olive oil is also a good source of vitamin K, the only richer sources being green leafy vegetables. Vitamin K is associated with the green pigment chlorophyll in olive oil. Vitamin K enables healthy blood clotting and aids our body's use of calcium, so encouraging strong bones, for example.

Polyphenols

Also known as phenolic compounds, these are olive oil's main antioxidants and many have potent antioxidant activity. The three main types are:

- *Phenols*, such as phenolic acids, tyrosol and oleuropeurin (see 'Scent and flavour compounds', page 29)

- *Secoiridoids*, such as oleocanthal (see 'Terpenes and terpenoids', page 28).

- *Lignans* – plant oestrogens, such as pinoresinol.

The levels of polyphenols in olive oil vary according to the method of cultivation, the amount of water in the soil, and the weather. Polyphenol levels in olive oil also vary with the:

- Variety of tree: for example, Koreneiki olives have high levels, Frantoio olives medium-high, Leccino olives medium and Arbequina olives low.

- Situation: altitude, latitude and type of soil of an olive farm.

- Ripeness of the olives: oil from green, unripe olives contains relatively high levels, which decline as the olives ripen.

- Production method: extra virgin and virgin olive oils contain the highest levels; adding water, churning, filtering, heating or using solvents lowers the levels.

- Storage conditions: the levels decrease as oxidation occurs in oil exposed to light, air or heat.

Olive oils possess different proportions of various polyphenols, according to the variety of olive. The more refined an olive oil, the lower is its concentration of polyphenols. For example, pinoresinol is virtually absent in refined olive oil. One tablespoon (about 12g) of extra virgin olive oil contains 7.5mg of polyphenols, so this oil is richer in polyphenols than are many other culinary oils. Of course, vegetables and fruits are vastly richer in polyphenols than are vegetable oils. Nevertheless, the amounts in extra virgin olive oil help make it a useful part of our diet. Researchers estimate that up to 65 per cent of the polyphenols we consume are absorbed from our digestive system intact.

Polyphenols help to make olive oil bitter. Their antioxidant and other properties mean that they aid health in a variety of ways. For example, the polyphenols in olive oil aid healing when applied to sunburned skin. They also help to lower raised blood pressure and are believed to help reduce high cholesterol and discourage heart attacks.

When we consume olive oil, its polyphenols help to prevent fats and cholesterol fermenting in our stomach and gut and are thought to encourage the production of fat-digesting enzymes in the pancreas.

Flavonoids and flavonols

The amounts of these antioxidant polyphenols in olive oil are small but worth having, as they help to:

- protect vitamin C by improving its absorption and protecting it from oxidation

- discourage heart attacks, strokes and certain other diseases

- strengthen the walls of capillaries (tiny blood vessels), so maximizing their potential volume and promoting good blood flow

- discourage cancer

The flavonol quercetin also has some anti-viral action.

Pigments

Carotenoids, chlorophyll and pheophytin are plant pigments responsible for the colour of different olive oils, which varies from light gold to deep olive or even emerald green. Their amounts and proportions determine an oil's colour. Green, unripe olives yield greener oil than do ripe olives because of their high chlorophyll content. Ripe olives are brown, reddish or black (depending on the variety) and yield yellow oil because they contain larger amounts of yellowish-red carotenoids (such as beta carotene). The presence of olive leaves during olive pressing makes the oil greener.

The amounts and proportions of pigments also depend on the type of olive tree, the soil, the weather and the extraction process. A deep colour is not necessarily a sign of high quality.

Fresh olive oil contains relatively more of the green pigment chlorophyll – though at up to 10 parts per million, this is nothing like the amount in spinach, for example. Some chlorophyll comes from olive leaves that enter the presses along with olives; certain producers encourage this to make their oil look greener. Chlorophyll is rich in magnesium, a mineral vital for every cell, particularly those in muscles, blood and nerves.

Chlorophyll acts as an antioxidant in olive oil that is protected from light. However, it is broken down during digestion, so has no antioxidant properties within our body.

Minerals

Very small amounts of certain minerals are present in olive oil. For example, it contains traces of calcium, chlorine, copper, iron, magnesium, manganese, phosphorus, selenium, sodium and zinc.

Terpenes and terpenoids

Olive oil contains an antioxidant terpenoid called squalene. This is present in unusually high concentrations in olive oil in comparison to other vegetable oils. Our body uses squalene to make cholesterol. Scientists believe that squalene is partially responsible for the health benefits of the Mediterranean Diet (see pages 32–3). They also suspect it may one day prove to help protect against cancer.

Another possible benefit from squalene is that by increasing the body's metabolic rate it supplies more oxygen to cells and therefore boosts our body's healing power. It may also promote liver function and bile secretion; enhance immunity; have anti-ageing, anti-fatigue, anti-bacterial and anti-inflammatory actions; improve vision; promote wound healing; and help to maintain normal alkalinity of the blood.

Organic acids and alcohols

The caffeic and gallic acids we consume in olive oil stimulate the release of bile from the gallbladder into the intestine. This helps to overcome the acidity of the food that has just left the stomach, enabling further digestion to occur in an alkaline environment.

An alcohol called phenylethanol in olive oil stimulates the production of fat-digesting enzymes in the pancreas. Also, a combination of this alcohol plus certain terpenes slows the absorption of cholesterol from food.

Sterols

Olive oil contains very small amounts of several sterols, including cholesterol, campesterol and beta-sitosterol. Some of these are useful to us – for example, beta-sitosterol is an antioxidant and also reduces the reabsorption of cholesterol excreted by our liver into our intestine.

Scent and flavour compounds

The antioxidant polyphenols oleuropein and oleocanthal help to give extra virgin olive oil a bitter peppery flavour. Oleocanthal has anti-inflammatory properties similar to those of non-steroidal anti-inflammatory drugs such as ibuprofen. The relatively large amounts in newly pressed extra virgin olive oil can make the throat sting.

The amounts of olive oil's various flavour constituents are determined by the variety of olive, the age of the olives at pressing, and the climate in which the trees are grown. The relatively cooler climatic conditions in Tuscany, for example, yield olives whose oil can often be described as fiery, whereas olive oils from warmer Mediterranean regions are frequently said to be sweeter and more buttery. Oils from the Peloponnese region in Greece have been described as green and grassy, with a slightly fiery finish, like that of a Tuscan oil. In addition, certain Italian oils are sometimes described as having the flavour of lemons, apples, new-mown hay, toasted nuts, chocolate or melon. Certain French oils taste fruity; and certain Spanish oils taste of almonds.

The amounts of olive oil's various flavour constituents are also influenced by the ripeness of the olives. Unripe olives produce more bitter or sharp-flavoured oil, while ripe olives produce 'sweeter' oil, and over-ripe olives produce oil that very quickly goes rancid. Roughly or otherwise badly processed oils also produce oil that quickly goes 'off'.

Other possible flavour descriptors of olive oils include, 'spicy', 'mild', 'tangy', 'pungent' and 'delicate'.

Although all olive oils have slight acidity, this is undetectable when we consume olive oil, because our taste receptors cannot detect acidity of below 6 per cent – and even that of the most acidic olive oil ('ordinary virgin olive oil') is only 3.3 per cent.

Peroxides

Air, light and heat oxidize olive oil's linoleic acid and fat-soluble vitamins such as vitamin E, forming peroxides, which smell and taste unpleasant and reduce the oil's nutritional content. The more oxidized the oil, the more peroxides are present and the more rancid it becomes.

Extra virgin olive oil must have a low peroxide level (less than 20 meq/kg). High-quality extra virgin olive oils have even lower levels (less than 10meq/kg).

Polycyclic aromatic hydrocarbons

Many foods naturally contain small quantities of polycyclic aromatic hydrocarbons (PAHs). Olive oil, like other vegetable oils, contains tiny amounts of up to 17 different PAHs, including benzanthracene and chrysene. Olive oil made from unripe olives generally contains more PAHs than that made from ripe ones.

Burning olive oil while cooking increases the amounts of PAHs, though the oil has to be heated repeatedly and for long periods to its smoking point for this to happen to any significant degree. Olive oil used for home cooking is unlikely ever to be a significant source of PAHs.

Microscopic fragments of olives

Tiny particles of olives contribute to the cloudy appearance of most extra virgin olive oils.

Contaminants

Traces of pesticides may be found in unrefined olive oils produced from olive farms that use herbicides and pesticides. Regulations in olive-producing and olive oil-importing countries should mean that only permitted pesticides are used and that any pesticide content in olive oil is within permitted limits. If you want to avoid using oil containing such pesticides, buy organic olive oil.

CHAPTER 4

Ailments and natural remedies

Neither olive oil nor monounsaturated fat is essential for the healthy working of the body. However, traditional use, common sense and anecdotal evidence suggest that olive oil as part of a healthy diet can help to prevent or treat many ailments. A large number of studies (some of them mentioned in this chapter) also provide scientific backing for these claims. The good balance of fats and the antioxidant content of olive oil help to explain why it promotes health.

An increasing amount of evidence associates olive oil (particularly as part of the Mediterranean Diet, which is relatively high in fat, mostly monounsaturated) with a lower risk of cardiovascular disease (heart attacks and strokes), obesity, metabolic syndrome, diabetes and high blood pressure. But such diseases are often more common in countries where a high fat intake results from animal fats, trans fats and polyunsaturated vegetable oils, such as corn oil.

Since I refer to the 'Mediterranean Diet' throughout this chapter, I'll explain here what the term means. The diet is based on the foods that were eaten in southern Italy and Crete in the 1960s, and contains minimally processed fresh vegetables, fruits, beans, nuts, seeds and grains. Small amounts of cheese and yogurt are eaten daily, fish and poultry weekly and no more than four eggs a week. Alcohol is consumed in moderation. Desserts, cakes and biscuits are eaten occasionally, and meat (mostly veal or lamb) about once a month. Vitamins, minerals, enzymes and antioxidants are plentiful. Olive oil is the main fat, so the fats are mostly monounsaturated, and saturated fats supply no more than 8 per cent of daily calories.

The dictionary of ailments in this chapter details how olive oil can help. However, please remember that:

- You can also discourage most ailments with a healthy diet, adequate hydration, regular exercise, daily outdoor light, effective stress management, a sensible alcohol intake and no smoking.

- The suggestions should not replace any necessary medical diagnosis and therapy.

- The amounts of olive oil recommended are for adults; a child would need less, depending on size.

- Added olive oil should take the place of other fat so as not to increase total daily calories.

- Olive oil should be consumed only as part of a healthy diet that is rich in whole foods, such as vegetables, fruits, whole grains and beans, and does not overload you with calories.

Whenever I suggest consuming olive oil in the rest of this chapter, you can do this in a variety of ways. For example, you can incorporate it into salad dressings, use it instead of butter on bread, fry with it, add it to certain cooked foods (such as pizzas) and use it instead of butter or other fat or oil in almost any recipe – unless its flavour would overwhelm that of the other ingredients.

When I mention a study, I give the journal's name and year of publication. These, plus some keywords, should enable you to discover more on the internet.

Acne

Olive oil can help because of its anti-bacterial and anti-inflammatory effects.

Action: Apply extra virgin olive oil to your skin two or three times a day.

Consume 2 tablespoons of extra virgin olive oil each day.

Age-related cognitive decline

Antioxidants such as those in extra virgin olive oil discourage memory loss and other cognitive decline. Scientists believe that monounsaturated fatty acids help by keeping brain-cell membranes healthy.

New York researchers put 1,393 people with normal cognitive ability on the Mediterranean Diet for 4½ years. During that time, 275 developed mild cognitive impairment. However, those of the 1,393 who adhered most closely to the diet were 28 per cent less likely to develop it than those who stuck to it least well. The researchers also put 482 people with pre-existing mild cognitive impairment on the same diet for 4½ years. During that time, 106 developed Alzheimer's disease.

However, those of the 482 who stuck most closely to the diet were only half as likely to develop Alzheimer's as those who stuck to it least well.

(*Archives of Neurology*, 2009)

In a study of elderly people in southern Italy, age-related cognitive decline was least likely in those who consumed most monounsaturated fat. The amount of olive oil consumed was inversely proportional to memory loss.

(*Journal of Nutrition*, 2008)

Action: Consume at least 2 tablespoons of extra virgin olive oil each day.

Age-related macular degeneration

This disease of an area at the back of the eye called the macula gradually destroys central vision and can eventually cause blindness. Olive oil may help to prevent it.

A study of women aged 50–79 associated higher intakes of monounsaturated fatty acid with a lower risk of AMD. In under-75s, total and saturated-fat intakes were associated with an increased risk.

(*Archives of Ophthalmology*, 2009)

In a study of 6,734 people aged 58–69, those who consumed at least 100ml (just over 3fl oz/scant ½ cup) of olive oil a week were less likely to get advanced AMD than those who consumed less than 1ml – meaning virtually no olive oil at all;

those who ate most trans-fats were the most likely to have advanced AMD; and those who ate most omega-3s were far less likely to have AMD.

(Archives of Ophthalmology, 2009)

Taking high-dose antioxidants and zinc reduces the risk of advanced AMD.

(Archives of Ophthalmology, 2001)

Action: Consume at least 2 tablespoons of extra virgin olive oil each day.

Alcohol intoxication

Some people believe that taking 1 tablespoon of olive oil before drinking alcohol helps to prevent a hangover.

Action: Try consuming 1 tablespoon of olive oil – either with food or on its own – before drinking alcohol.

Alzheimer's disease

This destroys brain cells and is associated with patches of amyloid protein and clusters of tangled nerve fibres. Experts believe that inflammation and damage from oxidation of brain fats are partly to blame.

Extra virgin olive oil's anti-inflammatory antioxidants counter oxidation and inflammation, and its monounsaturated fats help to keep brain-cell membranes healthy.

Researchers say that olive oil's oleocanthal binds to amyloid protein and reduces its damaging effects.

(Toxicology and Applied Pharmacology, 2009)

An overview of studies of over 1.5 million people found that strict adherence to the Mediterranean Diet cuts the risk of Alzheimer's by 13 per cent.

(British Medical Journal, 2008)

Laboratory tests in the US and Korea show that the antioxidant quercetin helps to protect rat brain cells from oxidation.

(Journal of Agricultural and Food Chemistry, 2004)

Action: Consume at least 2 tablespoons of extra virgin olive oil each day.

Arthritis

Inflammation is present in most arthritis. Olive oil can help, thanks to its antioxidants and monounsaturated fats. The antioxidant oleocanthal acts like the non-steroidal anti-inflammatory drug (NSAID) ibuprofen; and whereas long-term use of such a drug encourages intestinal bleeding and kidney damage, oleocanthal does not.

Research in Philadelphia shows that oleocanthal is an anti-inflammatory whose action (inhibition of COX-2 enzymes that enable prostaglandin formation) resembles that of the anti-inflammatory drug ibuprofen. Indeed, 2 tablespoons of olive oil have the same effect as 1/20th of the adult dose of ibuprofen.

(Nature, 2005)

Researchers report that olive oil's squalene, beta-sitosterol and tyrosol are antioxidants that discourage the production of inflammatory compounds from omega-6 fats (which we get mainly from red meat, corn oil and sunflower oil) or render them harmless.

(*Free Radical Biology and Medicine*, 2003)

A Greek study of 145 people with rheumatoid arthritis and 188 people without found that those with the lowest lifetime consumption of extra virgin olive oil and vegetables had a 2½ times greater risk of rheumatoid arthritis than those with the highest consumption. They suspect this is due to olive oil's antioxidants.

(*American Journal of Clinical Nutrition*, 1999)

Action: Consume 2 tablespoons of extra virgin olive oil each day. If your symptoms are bad, try consuming 4 tablespoons a day.

Asthma

This results from inflammation and oversensitivity of the airways. Consumption of olive oil has been associated with lower rates, possibly thanks to its monounsaturated fats, oleocanthal and other anti-inflammatories. Also, olive oil's quercetin acts as an antihistamine.

A study in Crete of nearly 700 children aged 7–18 shows that good adherence to the Mediterranean Diet helps to prevent asthma. Conversely, those who ate a lot of margarine had twice the risk.

(*Thorax*, 2006)

Research in Philadelphia shows that oleocanthal is an anti-inflammatory whose action (inhibition of COX-2 enzymes that enable prostaglandin formation) resembles that of the anti-inflammatory drug ibuprofen. Indeed, 2 tablespoons of olive oil have the same effect as 1/20th of the adult dose of ibuprofen. [See the comments about oleocanthal under 'Arthritis' on page 37.]

(*Nature*, 2005)

Action: To help prevent asthma, consume 2 tablespoons of extra virgin olive oil each day.

Burns

Applying olive oil to a small area of burnt skin can reduce pain and aid healing by keeping air from broken skin and by supplying antioxidants.

Action: Gently apply olive oil and repeat every hour or so.

Cancer

Cancer results from a mutation in a cell's genetic material (deoxyribonucleic acid, or DNA). Cancer cells continue multiplying instead of dying from apoptosis ('cell suicide') at their allotted time.

Research suggests that certain constituents of extra virgin olive oil help to prevent or treat certain cancers either because they reduce oxidation damage to DNA or because they influence hormones, immunity, cell-membrane composition or gene expression. Its antioxidants and anti-inflammatories, for example, may slow the development of cancer, encourage self-destruction of cancer cells and boost enzymes that block the activation of carcinogens and improve their removal from the body.

In particular:

- Polyphenols in virgin olive oil help to prevent bowel cancer.

- Lignans in olive oil have anti-cancer effects in the breasts, lung, skin and colon. Indeed, certain of these lignans are structurally similar to the breast-cancer drug tamoxifen.

- Polyphenols from pinoresinol-rich extra virgin olive oil have potent cancer-preventive properties.

- Polyphenols (especially secoiridoids and lignans) from extra virgin olive oil appear powerfully active against HER2-positive breast-cancer cells. Such cells test positive for a protein called human epidermal growth factor receptor 2 (HER2), which preomotes the growth of cancer cells. They tend to be more aggressive than other types of breast-cancer cell.

- Oleic acid (olive oil's main fatty acid) reduces the effect of an oncogene associated with rapid breast-cancer growth.

- Squalene, beta-sitosterol and tyrosol either inhibit oxidation of and production of inflammatory compounds from omega-6 fats (which we mainly get from red meat, corn oil and sunflower oil) or render them harmless.

Studies of more than 1.5 million people show that strict adherence to the Mediterranean Diet reduces the number of cancer deaths.

(*British Medical Journal*, 2008)

Bowel cancer

An olive oil-rich diet reduces the risk of bowel cancer, perhaps because it reduces the production of heterocyclic amines (HCAs) in meat as it cooks.

(Food Chemistry and Toxicology, 2003)

Making olive oil the main dietary fat seems to halve the risk of developing bowel cancer .

(American Journal of Medicine, 2002)

Olive oil promotes the replacement of cells in the bowel lining, which discourages cancer.

(Journal of Epidemiology and Community Health, 2000)

Consuming olive oil is associated with a lower cancer risk; eating a lot of meat with a higher risk. Researchers believe that a high meat intake boosts a bile acid, deoxycyclic acid, which dampens the activity of the enzyme diamine oxidase, which helps to regulate cell turnover in the bowel lining. Olive oil does the opposite, so protecting against abnormal cell growth and cancer.

Breast cancer

High adherence to the Mediterranean Diet, the main fat of which is olive oil, is associated with a slightly lower risk of breast cancer in over-50s.

(European Journal of Cancer, 2010)

Stomach cancer

High adherence to the Mediterranean Diet is associated with a reduced stomach-cancer risk.

(European Journal of Cancer, 2010)

Action: Consume at least 2 tablespoons of extra virgin olive oil each day.

Cataracts

Studies suggest that antioxidants help to prevent this clouding of the eye's lens, and a high intake of polyunsaturated fatty acids could be a risk factor. Extra virgin olive oil contains antioxidants; it's also much lower in polyunsaturated fatty acids than other common vegetable oils (such as sunflower and corn).

Data from the Harvard Nurses' Health Study indicates that a high intake of sunflower, corn, soya bean and cottonseed oils – which contain a high proportion of polyunsaturated fatty acids – is associated with a raised risk of cataracts.

(American Journal for Clinical Nutrition, 2005)

Action: Consume at least 2 tablespoons of extra virgin olive oil each day.

Chronic degenerative diseases

These include cardiovascular disease, diabetes, asthma and rheumatoid arthritis.

A high fat intake based on animal fats, corn and sunflower oil, and hydrogenated fats, is one of several risk factors. In contrast, a high fat intake in which olive oil is the main fat – such as with the Mediterranean

Diet – is associated with lower rates. This may be partly because the body uses olive oil's monounsaturated fats to produce substances that are relatively anti-inflammatory compared with the products of other fats. Olive oil also contains anti-inflammatory agents, including oleocanthal and squalene, which could aid prevention or treatment.

Research in Philadelphia shows that oleocanthal is an anti-inflammatory whose action (inhibition of COX-2 enzymes that enable prostaglandin formation) resembles that of the anti-inflammatory drug ibuprofen. Indeed, 2 tablespoons of olive oil have the same effect as 1/20th of the adult dose of ibuprofen.

(*Nature*, 2005)

Olive oil's squalene, beta-sitosterol and tyrosol are anti-oxidants that discourage production of inflammatory compounds from omega-6 fats (mainly found in meats, and corn and sunflower oils) or render them harmless.

(*Free Radical Biology and Medicine*, 2003)

Action: Consume 2 tablespoons of extra virgin olive oil each day.

Dandruff

This is often associated with infection by the fungus *Malassezia furfur*. Sometimes there is coexisting dermatitis (see 'Seborrhoeic dermatitis', page 71). Extra virgin olive oil's antifungal properties can help.

Action: Consume at least 2 tablespoons of extra virgin olive oil each day.

To treat dandruff, apply extra virgin olive oil to your scalp. Put a shower cap or plastic carrier bag over your hair and cover with a towel wrapped turban-style. Relax for 1 hour, then shampoo your hair. Repeat twice a week.

To prevent dandruff, use a home-made shampoo containing olive oil (see page 78).

Depression

Diet is one of several lifestyle factors that can either trigger or treat depression.

> A Spanish study of 10,094 healthy people found that those who followed the Mediterranean Diet most closely had a more than 30 per cent reduction in risk of depression compared with whose who adhered to it least well.
>
> (*Archives of General Psychiatry*, 2009)

Action: Consume at least 2 tablespoons of extra virgin olive oil each day.

Diabetes

With this condition, the pancreas makes little or none of the hormone insulin, so there is too much sugar in the blood but insufficient in the cells. High blood-sugar can damage arteries and veins; a lack of sugar in cells stops them functioning properly. The olive-oil-rich Mediterranean Diet helps to prevent and treat type 2 diabetes (the most common type).

In an Italian study of overweight adults with type 2 diabetes, one group ate a diet low in total and saturated fat, the other a Mediterranean Diet. All exercised and reduced their calorie intake. After the four years of the study, 56 per cent of the group on the Mediterranean Diet were able to control their blood sugar without medication, compared with 30 per cent of the low-fat group.

(*Annals of Internal Medicine*, 2009)

A Mediterranean Diet discourages type 2 diabetes, says a Spanish study of 13,380 people.

(*British Medical Journal*, 2008)

Action: Consume at least 2 tablespoons of extra virgin olive oil each day.

Ear wax

Olive oil can soften hard ear wax that is blocking the ear canal.

Action: Put one or two drops of warmed olive oil into the affected ear canal twice a day for a week.

Alternatively, soak a paper tissue in olive oil and warm it in the microwave. Squeeze warm oil from the tissue into your ear, then gently plug the ear with the tissue for an hour. Repeat daily for a week.

Eczema

Applying olive oil may help this dermatitis thanks to its anti-inflammatories such as squalene and other antioxidants. Consuming olive oil can help, too, as it has a relatively low ratio of omega-6 to omega-3 fatty acids, and eicosanoids (prostaglandins, leukotrienes, thromboxanes) made from omega-3s are less inflammatory than those made from omega-6s. Substances made in the body from olive oil's mono-unsaturated fats are also relatively less inflammatory than those made from polyunsaturated fats.

Action: Consume at least 2 tablespoons of extra virgin olive oil each day.

Smoothing extra virgin olive oil on your skin may help to ease irritation and prevent cracking.

Fainting

Feeling faint suggests that brain cells lack energy because of low blood sugar. Olive oil as part of a healthy diet may help to prevent this happening by keeping blood-sugar levels within a healthy range. Also, its squalene may help by increasing the metabolic rate and supplying more oxygen to cells.

Action: Consume at least 2 tablespoons of extra virgin olive oil each day.

Gallstones

Cholesterol-laden bile and a poorly contracting gallbladder encourage gallstones and are in turn encouraged by obesity, constipation and diabetes. Olive oil can help to prevent these diseases and may have other positive effects too.

Studies suggest that antioxidants discourage gallstones; olive oil is relatively rich in antioxidants.

Gallstones are more likely in over-acidic bile. Olive oil's slight acidity paradoxically discourages any tendency to unhealthy acidity in the body.

Olive oil's slight acidity encourages gallbladder contractions, helping to prevent the build-up of bile, which encourages gallstones.

A gallbladder flush (see below) aims to soften stones and encourage gallbladder contractions. Very few success stories have been verified by X-ray or scan, and the 'softened gallstones' reported in stools may just be lumps of actual soap made of bile salts and olive oil, but this treatment may be worth trying.

Action: Consume at least 2 tablespoons of extra virgin olive oil each day.

If you have stones, take 1 tablespoon each of olive oil and lemon juice 1 hour before breakfast each day.

Alternatively, consider a gallbladder flush (discussed first with your doctor). Drink 2 litres/3½ pints/8 cups of apple juice each day for 6 days. On the 7th day, miss supper; at 9pm, take 1–2 tablespoons of Epsom salts in a little water; at 10pm, drink 125ml/4fl oz/½ cup of olive oil shaken with 4 tablespoons of lemon juice, then lie on your left side for 30 minutes before bedtime.

Hair loss

Some people say that consuming olive oil and/or applying it to the scalp helps with this problem.

Action: Consume at least 2 tablespoons of extra virgin olive oil each day.

Also, apply extra virgin olive oil to your scalp, Put a shower cap or plastic carrier bag over your hair and cover with a towel wrapped turban-style. Relax for 1 hour, then rinse, shampoo and rinse again. Repeat twice a week.

Hay fever (allergic rhinitis)

Consuming olive oil may help to discourage the allergic inflammation of hay fever because some of its constituents are anti-inflammatory and its quercetin acts as an antihistamine.

> A study in Crete of nearly 700 children aged 7–18 suggests that the Mediterranean Diet (which includes olive oil) helps to prevent hay fever. Conversely, a high consumption of margarine is associated with double the risk.
>
> (*Thorax*, 2006)

Action: Consume at least 2 tablespoons of extra virgin olive oil each day.

Heart disease

Coronary artery disease begins when high blood pressure, cigarette-smoke toxins or high blood-fat or blood-sugar levels damage the arteries' lining (endothelium) and make it leak. LDL-cholesterol from blood can then seep into the artery walls, where it attracts white blood cells. These provoke inflammation, which oxidizes LDL-cholesterol; they then engulf the oxidized LDL-cholesterol and as a result swell into 'foam cells'. Calcium infiltrates the inflamed areas, and smooth-muscle cells produce collagen to cover the leaks. All this leads to atherosclerosis, with stiffened blood vessels and plaques of chalky fatty atheroma, which can rupture, encouraging clots that can trigger a heart attack.

Extra virgin olive oil, which is the main fat in the Mediterranean Diet, discourages oxidation, inflammation, high blood pressure, atherosclerosis and an unhealthy blood-fat profile (high LDL-cholesterol and triglycerides and low HDL-cholesterol). It also guards against diseases that encourage heart disease, such as obesity, high blood pressure and diabetes.

With olive oil the main dietary fat, oleic acid is the main fatty acid in both LDL- and HDL-cholesterol. This is good because oleic acid is more resistant than other fatty acids to oxidation. If extra virgin olive oil rather than refined olive oil is consumed, the oleic acid and other fats are further protected by polyphenols and other antioxidants.

Many other constituents of extra virgin olive oil are believed to be heart-protective too; these include:

- Anti-inflammatories: one of these, oleocanthal, has an action resembling that of the non-steroidal anti-inflammatory drug ibuprofen – 2 tablespoons of olive oil give the same effect as 1/20 of the adult dose of ibuprofen.

- Antioxidants, which discourage oxidation of LDL-cholesterol. Three antioxidants – squalene, beta-sitosterol and tyrosol – also discourage the production of inflammatory compounds from omega-6 fats, or render them harmless.

- Polyphenols, which help to prevent white blood cells sticking to the artery lining; one of them, hydroxytyrosol acetate, directly inhibits clotting.

Once olive oil's monounsaturated fatty acids have been absorbed from the intestine into the blood, they are either surrounded by protein molecules and thereby disguised as HDL- or LDL-cholesterol, or converted into other compounds. And all this takes place much more quickly than the 6–12 hours it would take to clear newly arrived saturated fatty acids from the blood. Scientists believe this speed of clearing fatty acids from the blood helps to prevent atherosclerosis. Olive oil's mono-unsaturated fats also help to prevent the blood from becoming sticky after a fatty meal and forming dangerous clots.

Indeed, the Food and Drug Administration in the United States allows olive-oil bottle labels to claim: 'Limited and not conclusive evidence suggests that eating about two tablespoons of olive oil daily may reduce the risk of coronary heart disease due to the monounsaturated fat in olive oil.' However, labels must also say: 'To achieve this possible benefit, olive oil is to replace a similar amount of saturated fat and not increase the total number of calories you eat in a day.'

Please note, however, that increasing numbers of studies suggest that provided we don't overeat, neither a high total intake of fat nor a high intake of saturated fats should be considered a risk factor for heart disease. What seems more important is what we *should* eat rather than what we should *not* eat.

A study of about 30,000 Italian women found those who consumed at least 3 tablespoons of olive oil a day had nearly half the risk of heart disease compared with those who consumed less.

(American Journal of Clinical Nutrition, 2010)

An overview of 21 studies involving 348,000 people found no relationship between saturated-fat intake and heart attacks.

(Archives of Internal Medicine, 2010)

A Spanish study of 13,609 people found that those with the highest adherence to the Mediterranean Diet had a lower heart-disease risk than those with the lowest adherence.

(Nutrition, Metabolism and Cardiovascular Diseases, 2010)

An overview of 12 studies, involving over 1.5 million people, found that strict adherence to the Mediterranean Diet reduces the risk of dying from a heart attack or a stroke by 9 per cent.

(British Medical Journal, 2008)

Making olive oil the only added dietary fat nearly halves the risk of coronary heart disease, according to a Greek study of 1,926 people.

(Clinical Cardiology, 2007)

Extra virgin olive oil is best for heart health, reports a study in which 200 men used 5 teaspoons of refined, virgin or extra virgin olive oil (containing, respectively, low, medium and high levels of polyphenols) to replace the equivalent amount of their usual dietary fat each day. Their HDL-cholesterol level was highest with extra virgin olive oil and lowest with refined olive oil. In contrast, their LDL-cholesterol was lowest with extra virgin olive oil and highest with refined olive oil. The ratio of total cholesterol to HDL-cholesterol, and the oxidation of LDL-cholesterol, decreased with oils of increasing polyphenol content.

(Annals of Internal Medicine, 2006)

A study of almost 49,000 women reports almost identical rates of heart attacks in women who followed a low-fat diet and those who did not.

(Journal of the American Medical Association, 2006)

Participants in this study ate breakfasts of bread and either extra virgin olive oil or refined olive oil. After a breakfast containing extra virgin olive oil (which has a relatively high polyphenol content), their arteries became more elastic. But after a breakfast containing olive oil (which has a low polyphenol content) there was no change in their usual arterial elasticity.

(International Journal of Vitamin and Nutrition Research, 2005)

This study shows that adding 2 tablespoons of extra virgin olive oil to the daily diet lowers total cholesterol, LDL-cholesterol and omega-6 fatty acid levels.

(Medical Science Monitor, 2004)

People who consume 2 tablespoons of virgin olive oil a day have less oxidation of their LDL-cholesterol and higher antioxidant levels than people who consume smaller amounts, or none at all.

(European Journal of Clinical Nutrition, 2002)

In the Nurses' Health Study of 80,082 women, substituting 80 calories of monounsaturated or polyunsaturated fat for 80 calories of carbohydrate lowered the heart-disease risk by 30 to 40 per cent. The total fat intake was unrelated to risk; trans-fat intake raised it.

(New England Journal of Medicine, 1997)

Action: Consume at least 2 tablespoons of extra virgin olive oil each day.

High blood pressure

Risk factors for high blood pressure include obesity (partly because more body tissue means more work for the heart) and atherosclerosis (see 'Heart disease'). Olive-oil consumption discourages both. Also, its polyphenols and magnesium may help. Note that adding olive oil to your diet while on high-blood-pressure medication might lower your blood pressure enough to make your current dose of medication too high. So monitor your blood pressure and if necessary discuss with your doctor whether to change the dose.

A high-carbohydrate diet, a high-protein diet, and a diet high in monounsaturated fat (thanks to olive oil, canola oil or olive-oil spread) found that all the diets reduced blood pressure and total and LDL-cholesterol levels.

(Journal of the American Dietetics Association, 2008)

Adding 5 teaspoons of olive oil each day (in place of an equivalent amount of other fat) to the diet reduced men's systolic blood pressure by 3 per cent (a small but potentially useful amount).

(Journal of Nutrition, 2007)

A Greek study of more than 20,000 people eating the Mediterranean Diet associated extra virgin olive oil and vegetables with lower blood pressure, and cereals, meat and alcohol with higher blood pressure. Olive oil was the main factor in lowering blood pressure, probably thanks to its poly-phenols rather than its monounsaturated fats.

(American Journal of Clinical Nutrition, 2004)

A Spanish study reports that the blood pressure of women with high blood pressure fell when they added olive oil to their diet. In contrast, adding a type of sunflower oil rich in oleic acid had no effect. This suggests that components of olive oil other than its monounsaturated fat are responsible.

(Journal of Hypertension, 1996)

Action: Consume at least 2 tablespoons of extra virgin olive oil each day.

High cholesterol

See Chapter 3 for more information on cholesterol. An unhealthy diet, a lack of exercise and insufficient sunlight encourage high LDL-cholesterol, high total cholesterol, and low HDL-cholesterol in the body. Smoking, stress and an unhealthy diet encourage oxidation of LDL-cholesterol. Oxidized LDL encourages high blood pressure, cardiovascular disease (heart attacks and strokes) and several other diseases.

For most people, the liver makes 80 per cent of their cholesterol, and dietary cholesterol is only a minor source. For some, though, dietary cholesterol is more important, and avoiding cholesterol-rich foods has a bigger effect on cholesterol levels. No test can currently identify this group.

It is wrong to call LDL-cholesterol 'bad' cholesterol, since only when it is oxidized does it encourage cardiovascular disease. However, calling HDL-cholesterol 'good' cholesterol *is* appropriate because the higher it is, the lower the risk of cardiovascular disease. Scientists estimate HDL-cholesterol's ability to predict coronary heart disease as being four times greater than that of LDL-cholesterol and eight times greater than that of total cholesterol. An HDL-cholesterol level of 60 mg/dl (1.56 mmol/l) or more is considered protective against heart disease. Note, though, that certain rural-living people in Japan not only have the world's lowest rate of heart disease but also have very low HDL-cholesterol – so other protective factors (perhaps including a high oily-fish intake, other dietary factors, low alcohol intake, exercise and low weight) can clearly be more important.

The ratio of total cholesterol to HDL-cholesterol is another important indicator of heart-disease risk, as shown overleaf.

In the US, India and many other countries, cholesterol levels are reported in mg/dl, and in Europe and Australia in mmol/l. To convert mmol/l of glucose to mg/dl, multiply by 18; to convert mg/dl to mmol/l, divide by 18.

Several olive-oil constituents, including fatty acids and polyphenols and other antioxidants, have beneficial effects on cholesterol production and metabolism. Also, its sitosterol reduces

HEART-DISEASE RISK IMPLIED BY THE RATIO OF TOTAL CHOLESTEROL TO HDL-CHOLESTEROL

Risk	Total:HDL ratio in men	Total:HDL ratio in women
Very low	less than 3.4	Less than 3.3
Low	4.0	3.8
Average	5.0	4.5
Moderate	9.5	7.0
High	more than 23	more than 11

the intestinal absorption of dietary cholesterol. If you take statins for high cholesterol, note that consuming olive oil may lower your cholesterol, so have it checked in case you should lower the dose.

A study of diets high in carbohydrate, protein or unsaturated fat (from olive oil, canola oil and olive oil spread – each rich in monounsaturated fat) found that each reduced total cholesterol and LDL-cholesterol.

(*Journal of the American Dietetics Association*, 2008)

Consuming olive oil improved the fatty-acid profile of LDL-cholesterol and reduced oxidation of LDL-cholesterol.

(*Journal of the American College of Nutrition*, 2008)

Consuming extra virgin olive oil (which is rich in clot-fighting phenols) discourages clots (such as those causing heart attacks and strokes) after a meal in people with high cholesterol.

(*American Journal of Clinical Nutrition*, 2007)

Researchers report that the higher an olive oil's polyphenol content, the higher the resulting increase in HDL-cholesterol. The ratio of total cholesterol to HDL-cholesterol, and the degree of oxidation of LDL-cholesterol, decreased with increasing polyphenolic content.

(*Annals of Internal Medicine*, 2006)

Dutch researchers analysed 60 trials of the effects of carbohydrates and fats on blood lipids. In those in which polyunsaturated and monounsaturated fats were eaten in place of carbohydrates, LDL-cholesterol decreased and HDL-cholesterol increased.

(*Journal of the American Medical Association*, 2005)

When 21 volunteers with a high cholesterol level ate a breakfast containing virgin olive oil, their blood contained far fewer free radicals than normal after a meal. But when they ate breakfast containing olive oil with a lower polyphenol concentration, the beneficial effects were virtually absent.

(*Journal of the American College of Cardiology*, 2005)

Action: Consume at least 2 tablespoons of extra virgin olive oil each day.

Indigestion

Olive oil stimulates the production of bile in the liver and its expulsion from the gallbladder into the intestine, so as part of a healthy diet it can help to prevent indigestion caused by the poor digestion of fats.

Action: Consume 1–2 tablespoons of extra virgin olive oil with each fatty meal.

Infection

Extra virgin olive oil, whether consumed or applied to the skin, has some antibacterial, antiviral and antifungal activity, thanks to its polyphenols and other antioxidants.

> An extract of virgin olive oil added to mayonnaise or salad inoculated with salmonella and listeria bacteria reduced the bacterial counts. The researchers attribute this to olive oil's polyphenols and believe that olive oil could help to protect against gastroenteritis from contaminated food.
>
> *(Journal of Food Protection, 2007)*

Action: Consume at least 2 tablespoons of extra virgin olive oil each day.

Inflammation

Many constituents of olive oil are anti-inflammatory – including squalene, beta-sitosterol, tyrosol, oleocanthal and monounsaturated fatty acids. This may explain its potential benefit in diseases that involve inflammation, including Alzheimer's, arthritis, asthma, diabetes, eczema, hay fever, heart disease, infection, inflammatory bowel disease, metabolic syndrome, psoriasis and strokes.

Research in Philadelphia shows that oleocanthal is an anti-inflammatory whose action (inhibition of COX-2 enzymes that enable prostaglandin formation) resembles that of the anti-inflammatory drug ibuprofen. Indeed, 2 tablespoons of olive oil have the same effect as 1/20th of the adult dose of ibuprofen.

(*Nature*, 2005)

Action: Consume 2 tablespoons of extra virgin olive oil each day.

Inflammatory bowel disease

Powerful drugs such as steroids can dampen the symptoms of ulcerative colitis and Crohn's disease, but there is no cure. However, one piece of good news is that olive oil may help to prevent ulcerative colitis.

In a study of more than 25,000 people, none with ulcerative colitis at first, those with the highest oleic-acid intake had a 90 per cent lower risk of developing it. The researchers suspect that oleic acid helps to prevent ulcerative colitis by blocking inflammatory chemicals in the bowel. They estimate that one in two cases could be prevented by consuming 2–3 tablespoons of olive oil a day, and say that future research should assess oleic acid as a possible treatment.

(Presented at the Digestive Disease Week conference in New Orleans, 2010)

Action: Consume at least 2 tablespoons of extra virgin olive oil a day.

Metabolic syndrome

At least a quarter of the world's population is said to have metabolic syndrome. The diagnosis turns on having at least three of the following:

- Insulin resistance

- High blood pressure

- High blood fats

- Low HDL-cholesterol

- An apple-shaped abdomen

A woman is probably apple-shaped and her health at risk if her waist measures 32in (80cm) or more. Her risk is greater if her waist is 35in (88cm) or more.

A man's health is at risk if his waist is 37in (94cm) or more. His risk is greater with a waist of 40in (102cm) or more.

Metabolic syndrome is encouraged by a lack of exercise and an unhealthy diet (with a poor balance of fats and too much refined carbohydrate – such as sugar and white flour). It greatly encourages diabetes, heart disease and strokes.

Olive oil as part of a healthy diet may help to prevent it because, for example, of the effects of its polyphenols, squalene and mono-unsaturated fat.

A study of 20 people with metabolic syndrome found changes in genes whose activity is regulated by olive-oil poly-phenols. Virgin olive oil suppressed 98 genes, many of them linked to obesity, high blood fats, diabetes and heart disease, and several concerned with pro-inflammatory processes. The researchers suggest that olive oil can 'switch off' certain genes that control immune cells, so these are less likely to induce inflammation.

(BMC Genomics, 2010)

A study of 808 people at high risk of cardiovascular disease found that adherence to the Mediterranean Diet discouraged metabolic syndrome. Those with the highest adherence were half as likely to have low HDL-cholesterol and high triglycerides compared with those with lowest adherence.

(Nutrition, Metabolism and Cardiovascular Disease, 2009)

Action: Consume at least 2 tablespoons of extra virgin olive oil each day.

Nappy (diaper) rash

Olive oil can reasonably be expected to soothe inflammation from nappy (diaper) dermatitis.

Action: Smooth a little extra virgin olive oil over the inflamed skin after cleaning the skin during each nappy change.

Obesity

A high consumption of fat often used to be blamed for obesity, but these statistics show this cannot be so. In the 1960s, Americans obtained 45 per cent of their calories from fats, and 13 per cent were obese. But in 2010, Americans obtained only 33 per cent of their calories from fats, yet 34 per cent were obese.

Of course, fat can contribute to obesity if your diet contains too many calories. But you can eat any amount of fat without it making you fat, if this fits into a healthy balanced diet and provides necessary calories.

There are several reasons why olive oil as part of a healthy diet could help to prevent or treat obesity, or discourage related diseases:

- Including olive oil (or other fat) in each meal stimulates the release of the hormone cholecystokinin, which helps to suppress hunger.

- Olive oil's slight acidity, provided it is not neutralized by other foods, can slow sugar absorption, keeping your blood-sugar level steadier for longer and helping to prevent hunger and therefore overeating between meals.

- Acidic foods help to compensate for any lack of stomach acid (which affects one in two over-60s). Low stomach acid leads to poor absorption of protein and certain other nutrients, which can encourage hunger and overeating. Olive oil is only slightly acidic but it helps a little.

- Olive oil's omega-3 polyunsaturated fats 'switch on' fat-burning genes.

- Olive oil partially inhibits stomach contractions. This means the stomach's contents empty more slowly after a meal, which prolongs the feeling of fullness.

- Obesity encourages inflammation in various parts of the body; extra virgin olive oil contains several anti-inflammatory agents.

- Olive oil's oleuropein may encourage weight loss by boosting the body's heat production and thus its use of calories.

- Food fried in olive oil has a lower fat content than food fried in other oils, because olive oil has a higher smoke point. This means it can be heated to a higher temperature. In addition, a relatively high frying temperature creates a crust on the surface of the food, which prevents it soaking up a lot of oil.

- As when using any culinary oil, heat olive oil in the pan before you add the food to be fried, since food put into cold oil soaks it up, which increases its calorie content.

A Spanish study of 613 people found that the consumption of olive oil (which is rich in monounsaturated fat) reduced the risk of obesity compared with the consumption of sunflower oil (rich in polyunsaturated fat).

(*European Journal of Clinical Nutrition*, 2009)

A Japanese study in rats found that oleuropein decreased body weight. It did this by encouraging a particularly meta-bolically active type of body fat called brown fat to burn calories, and also by encouraging the production of the hormones noradrenaline and adrenaline.

(*Journal of Nutritional Science and Vitaminology*, 2008)

Olive oil contains a monounsaturated fat called oleic acid. When olive oil is consumed, cells in the small intestine convert oleic acid into a substance called oleoylethanolamide, which curbs hunger.

(*Cell Metabolism*, 2008)

> Substituting olive oil for saturated fat in the diet was associated with a small loss of body weight and fat mass.
>
> *(British Journal of Nutrition, 2003)*

Action: Consume at least 2 tablespoons of extra virgin olive oil each day as part of a healthy diet that provides the calories needed to maintain your goal weight.

Osteoporosis

A Western woman's lifetime risk of a fracture from this bone-thinning condition is 30–40 per cent, a man's about 13 per cent. Osteoporosis risk factors include a poor diet, obesity, age, over-exercising and smoking. Research suggests that inflammation and oxidation play an important part, and olive oil as part of a healthy diet might help for the following reasons:

- Extra virgin olive oil contains a variety of antioxidants and anti-inflammatory agents.

- Olive oil aids calcium absorption.

- Increased olive oil consumption is associated with increased bone mineralization.

- Good bone mineralization is dependent on consuming enough oleic acid (the main fatty acid in olive oil) and essential fatty acids.

- The Mediterranean Diet discourages osteoporosis.

Studies at the National Institute for Agricultural Research in France show that two olive-oil polyphenols – oleuropein and hydroxytyrosol – greatly reduce inflammation-induced bone loss in osteoporosis. (So dramatic is this effect that the Belgian firm BioActor has patents to use these polyphenols in foods, food supplements and herbal medicines for osteo-porosis prevention.)

(Osteoporosis International, 2010)

The lowest incidence of osteoporosis in Europe is around the Mediterranean. The beneficial effect is attributed mainly to the diet.

(Médecine Science, 2007)

Action: Consume at least 2 tablespoons of extra virgin olive oil each day.

Pain

It is possible that oleocanthal in extra virgin olive oil might help to ease pain caused by inflammation.

Research in Philadelphia shows that oleocanthal is an anti-inflammatory whose action (inhibition of COX-2 enzymes that enable prostaglandin formation) resembles that of the anti-inflammatory drug ibuprofen. Indeed, 2 tablespoons of olive oil have the same effect as 1/20th of the adult dose of ibuprofen.

(Nature, 2005)

Action: Consume at least 2 tablespoons of extra virgin olive oil each day.

Parkinson's disease

Scientists suspect that strict adherence to the Mediterranean Diet – of which olive oil is an important part – is associated with a lower risk of this disease.

> An overview of 12 studies involving more than 1.5 million people shows that strict adherence to the Mediterranean Diet is associated with a 13 per cent reduction in risk of Parkinson's disease.
>
> (*British Medical Journal*, 2008)

Action: Consume at least 2 tablespoons of extra virgin olive oil each day.

Peptic ulcer

An ulcer can develop if something interferes with the stomach's protective mucus, lining or acid. It is a common misconception that people with ulcers make too much acid: in fact, most don't, and many make too little. Inflammation caused by an infection with *Helicobacter pylori* bacteria is a major cause of not only peptic ulcers but also stomach inflammation (gastritis) and cancer. Unfortunately, *Helicobacter pylori* bacteria are becoming increasingly resistant to antibiotics. The good news is that olive oil may help.

A Spanish study involving test-tube experiments reveals that polyphenols diffuse from olive oil into stomach acid, where they exert strong activity against *Helicobacter pylori* (even antibiotic-resistant types) for several hours. One polyphenol, Ty-EDA, was so effective that only 1.5 μg/ml was needed to kill the bacteria. To put this into perspective, most virgin olive oils contain up to 240 μg/ml of Ty-EDA. The researchers note that the concentration of olive-oil polyphenols needed to kill bacteria was much lower than the necessary concentrations of polyphenols from tea and wine would have been.

(Journal of Agriculture and Food Chemistry, 2007)

A Russian study found that when people with a peptic ulcer replaced animal fat in their diet with olive oil, the ulcer's size greatly decreased and healing improved.

(Vrachebnoe delo, 1986)

Action: Consume at least 2 tablespoons of extra virgin olive oil each day.

Polycystic ovary syndrome

This condition is characterized by some combination of obesity, irregular or absent periods, infertility, acne, excess facial and bodily hair, and thinning hair on temples and crown, plus 10 or more cysts on each ovary. Without treatment, the menopause is usually early and the risk of diabetes, high blood pressure, strokes and womb cancer is increased. It often begins after suddenly gaining weight or stopping oral contraception, and can run in families.

Insensitivity to insulin (a hormone that regulates blood sugar and fat metabolism) is common and associated with eating too much high-glycaemic-index (blood-sugar-raising) food. Insulin resistance eventually leads to high blood levels of insulin – which researchers think is the key factor.

> An Italian study shows that substituting olive oil for saturated fat in the diet helps to lower blood sugar.
>
> (*Diabetologia*, 2001)

Action: Consume at least 2 tablespoons of extra virgin olive oil each day.

Poor circulation

The factors that encourage cardiovascular disease (see 'Heart disease' and 'Strokes') also encourage poor circulation. So olive oil as part of a healthy diet may help.

Action: Consume at least 2 tablespoons of extra virgin olive oil each day.

Poor libido

There's a saying in Greece: 'Eat butter and sleep tight, eat olive oil and come at night'. Certainly, folklore suggests that olive oil has aphrodisiac properties.

Action: Try consuming 1 tablespoon of extra virgin olive oil in the early evening.

Premature ageing

Damage by excessive oxidation encourages premature ageing. This is more likely in people who smoke, eat an unhealthy diet or are stressed. Extra virgin olive oil's monounsaturated fat and antioxidants help to prevent excessive oxidation. One particular antioxidant, squalene, may have an additional anti-ageing benefit because it increases metabolism, thus supplying more oxygen to cells.

It is said that in Lebanon there is a village where the people drink a glass of olive oil morning and evening; their average lifespan is 98 for the women and 97 for the men.

US researchers say that mineral and vitamin deficiencies speed the age-related decay of the cells' mitochondria (energy-providing structures).

(Molecular Aspects of Medicine, 2005)

Australian research suggests that people with a high intake of vegetables and olive oil, but a low intake of dairy products, margarine and sugar, had the youngest looking skin.

(Journal of the American College of Nutrition, 2001)

Action: Consume at least 2 tablespoons of extra virgin olive oil each day.

Premature death

The Mediterranean Diet, which contains olive oil, seems to help prevent premature death.

An overview of 12 studies involving more than 1.5 million
people found that strict adherence to the Mediterranean Diet
cut the risk of all-cause early death by 9 per cent.

(British Medical Journal, 2008)

A 6-year study of 5,611 over-60s associated the
Mediterranean Diet with a 50 per cent reduction in risk of
dying during the study. The researchers concluded: 'Dietary
recommendations aimed at the Italian elderly population
should support a dietary pattern characterized by a high consumption of olive oil, raw vegetables and poultry.'

(British Journal of Nutrition, 2007)

Action: Consume at least 2 tablespoons of extra virgin olive oil
each day.

Psoriasis

Psoriasis is characterized by patches of thick, flaking skin overlying
inflammation on the knees, elbows, scalp or elsewhere.

Applying or consuming olive oil may soothe the inflammation,
thanks to anti-inflammatory constituents such as monounsaturated
fats, and oleocanthal and other antioxidants.

Research in Philadelphia shows that oleocanthal is an anti-
inflammatory whose action (inhibition of COX-2 enzymes
that enable prostaglandin formation) resembles that of the
anti-inflammatory drug ibuprofen. Indeed, 2 tablespoons of
olive oil have the same effect as 1/20th of the adult dose of
ibuprofen.

(Nature, 2005)

Action: Consume at least 2 tablespoons of extra virgin olive oil each day.

To help treat psoriasis, apply a thin film of extra virgin olive oil to affected skin twice a day.

Scars

It is said that applying olive oil to healing scars, including stretch marks, can reduce the eventual scarring.

Action: Apply extra virgin olive oil to healing scars each day.

Seborrhoeic dermatitis

This is a type of skin inflammation that affects areas with the most sebaceous glands, such as the scalp, behind the ears, between the eyebrows, along the eyelashes and around the nose. It is often caused by an overgrowth of yeasts called *Malassezia furfur* that are normal skin inhabitants. Many people with this condition also have dandruff (see pages 43–4).

Extra virgin olive oil makes a gentle cleanser, has antifungal properties and softens scaly areas.

Action: Smooth extra virgin olive oil into the affected skin twice a day. If your scalp is affected, apply extra virgin olive oil. Put a shower cap or plastic carrier bag over your hair and cover with a towel wrapped turban-style. Relax for 1 hour, then shampoo your hair. Repeat twice a week.

Consume at least 2 tablespoons of extra virgin olive oil each day.

Strokes

Most strokes ('brain attacks') are 'thrombotic', resulting from a clot interrupting the blood flow in a brain artery. The main culprit is atherosclerosis (see 'Heart disease'), which roughens and inflames arteries and makes them narrow and stiff. Clots readily form in atherosclerotic arteries, especially if there are other risk factors such as smoking, stress, an unhealthy diet, obesity, high blood pressure, diabetes, chronic infection or an unhealthy cholesterol balance. Making extra virgin olive oil the main fat in your diet can help to counter many of the risk factors for atherosclerosis.

A study of the medical history of 7,625 people aged 65 and over, from Bordeaux, Dijon and Montpellier, in France, over 5 years, reported that those who regularly used olive oil in their cooking or with bread or as a dressing had a 41% lower risk of a stroke than those who never consumed it.

(Neurology, 2011)

A Spanish study of 13,609 people initially free from cardiovascular disease found that those with the highest adherence to the Mediterranean Diet had a smaller risk of strokes than those with the lowest adherence.

(Nutrition, Metabolism and Cardiovascular Diseases, 2010)

An overview of 12 studies involving more than 1.5 million people found that strict adherence to the Mediterranean Diet cuts the risk of dying from a stroke or a heart attack by 9 per cent.

(British Medical Journal, 2008)

Doctors sometimes recommend low-dose aspirin to discourage a stroke, partly because of its anti-inflammatory and anti-blood-clotting actions. This study tested one of the polyphenols in virgin olive oil, hydroxytyrosol acetate, and found that it inhibited clotting. So it is possible that consuming olive oil as part of a healthy diet, and along with any medically recommended treatment, might help prevent a thrombotic stroke.

(*British Journal of Nutrition*, 2008)

A review at Boston University suggests that flavonoids (such as those in olive oil) help to prevent blood clots by making artery walls more flexible.

(*American Journal of Clinical Nutrition*, 2005)

Action: Consume at least 2 tablespoons of extra virgin olive oil each day.

Warts

Olive oil's flavonoids can stop wart viruses from multiplying.

Action: Consume at least 2 tablespoons of extra virgin olive oil each day to help prevent warts.

To treat a wart, apply extra virgin olive oil to the wart, then cover the wart with a sticking plaster (adhesive bandage). Repeat twice a day for 3–6 weeks.

CHAPTER 5

Beauty aid

The ancient Greeks cleansed and moisturized their skin with olive oil, and over the millennia this oil has been used not only directly on the skin but also to make a variety of beauty products – including soaps, shower gels, exfoliating scrubs, shampoos, moisturizers, hand creams, moisturizing 'dry' oils, nail oils, lip balms, massage oils and after-sun soothing creams.

Applying olive oil to the skin helps to prevent moisture loss, soothes inflammation, has some antimicrobial effect and confers a lovely soft sheen. Most importantly, its slight acidity means that it is gentle compared with some commercial toiletries, such as most soaps (see below).

Normal skin is coated with a slightly acidic surface layer called the 'acid mantle' or 'hydro-lipid film'. This contains:

- Fats (lipids) from skin oil (sebum)

- Lactic acid and amino acids from sweat

- Amino acids and pyrrolidine carboxylic acid from dead skin cells.

The acidity of the skin's surface layer and of water-soluble toiletries is measured in terms of their pH (hydrogen ion concentration). Below 7 is acidic, 7 is neutral, above 7 is alkaline. The further below 7 the pH is, the more acidic the liquid, whereas the further above 7 the pH is, the more alkaline it is.

In women, the skin's normal pH over most of the body is 4.5–5.75; in men it is marginally more acidic. This slight acidity helps to repair damaged skin and activates enzymes that enable the production of lipids in sebum. Intact skin and healthy sebum help to prevent water escaping from the skin (other than in perspiration) and harmful substances and micro-organisms entering it. The slight acidity also promotes normal-sized populations of skin-friendly bacteria and fungi and helps to prevent infection. Any reduction in skin acidity – caused, for example, by using most soaps (which are alkaline) or if you have dermatitis – encourages drying, cracking and itching.

Olive oil, like other vegetable oils, is weakly acidic, so applying it to the skin does not compromise normal skin acidity as much as most soaps. Since oil is insoluble in water, its acidity cannot be measured as pH (see below). Instead, acidity is calculated as the percentage of free fatty acids in the oil. Better-quality oils are less acidic, poorer-quality oils more acidic. According to the International Olive Council's regulations, extra virgin olive oil must have less than 0.8 per cent free fatty acid; some refined olive oils have less than 0.1 per cent.

Extra virgin olive oil also contains many skin-friendly substances, including antioxidants (which help to protect sebum from oxidation), anti-inflammatories (monounsaturated fat and antioxidants) and anti-microbials (such as polyphenols).

All in all, olive oil softens, moisturizes and soothes skin, helps to maintain its elasticity and helps to counter infection. It gives nails an attractive sheen and softens and nourishes the cuticles. It also conditions hair and makes it shine. You can use it at home to make a variety of excellent beauty products. Store any surplus in the refrigerator for up to a week, and let it come to room temperature before using it.

Eye makeup remover

To remove eye makeup, pour a little extra virgin olive oil on to a cotton-wool ball (cotton pad) and smooth this over your eyelids.

Exfoliating scrub

Mix 1 tablespoon of caster sugar with enough extra virgin olive oil to make a firm paste. Rub this on to your skin until the sugar dissolves, then rinse off with warm water.

Moisturizer

Apply extra virgin olive oil to help prevent moisture loss from your skin and to soften it and give it a sheen.

To make a soothing, softening moisturizing cream, put 1 tablespoon of beeswax into a basin and melt it by standing the basin in the top of a double boiler or a *bain marie*, or directly in a pan containing enough boiling water to come no more than half way up the basin. Beat in 3 tablespoons of extra virgin olive oil. Remove from the heat and beat in 1 teaspoon of apple cider vinegar and 2 teaspoons of water. Stir until the cream is lukewarm, then stir in 3 drops of an essential oil, choosing from chamomile, frankincense, lavender, neroli, rose, sandalwood or ylang ylang, all of which are fragrant and have skin-regenerating properties. Apply to your skin.

For a soothing, moisturizing milk for your skin, put into a bowl 2 tablespoons of extra virgin olive oil, 2 teaspoons of clear honey, 1 teaspoon of apple cider vinegar and 1 tablespoon of full-fat plain bio yoghurt, and mix well. Apply with a cotton-wool ball (cotton pad).

To soften dry skin on your elbows or feet, gently massage in a small amount of olive oil.

Face mask

Make a moisturizing, soothing and rejuvenating mask by putting into a small bowl 1 tablespoon of extra virgin olive oil, 1 tablespoon of clear honey, 1 tablespoon of plain full-fat bio-yoghurt and 1 egg yolk. Mix well. Apply this mask to your face, then relax for 30 minutes before rinsing off with warm water.

Bath oil

For a fragrant bath oil, add 2 tablespoons of extra virgin olive oil and 6 drops of essential oil (such as geranium, neroli or lavender) to the tap water as it runs into your bath. Take care in the bath, as the oil will make it slippery.

Hair-treatment oil

Put 3 tablespoons of extra virgin olive oil into a small bowl, then pour the oil over your hair and gently rub it in. Put a shower cap or plastic carrier bag over your hair and cover with a towel wrapped turban-style. Relax for 30 minutes then shampoo your hair.

Shampoo

Put 2 tablespoons of olive oil, 1 egg, 1 tablespoon of lemon juice, and ½ teaspoon of apple cider vinegar into a bowl, blend with a fork or small whisk and use as normal shampoo.

Nail and cuticle oil

Put into an eggcup 1 teaspoon of extra virgin olive oil and 1 drop of frankincense, lemon or neroli essential oil. Stir the fragrant oil, then gently rub it on to your fingernails and toenails.

Lip balm

Put 2 tablespoons of beeswax into a basin and stand it in a pan of boiling water until the beeswax melts. Remove from the heat and leave to cool, then stir in 4 tablespoons of olive oil, 3 drops of an essential oil (such as lavender or chamomile) and 2 teaspoons of honey. Apply to your lips as necessary.

Smooth extra virgin olive oil directly on to dry or sore lips to soothe and soften them or to help them to heal.

Massage oil

Put into a small bowl or bottle 2 tablespoons of extra virgin olive oil and 10 drops of one or more fragrant essential oils. (Cedarwood, frankincense and lavender oils are said to be relaxing; geranium, jasmine, neroli and ylang ylang uplifting; and cardamom stimulating.) Mix the oils well before use.

CHAPTER 6

Choosing and using olive oil

Extra virgin olive oil is the best olive oil for odour, flavour, nutrient value, health-giving properties and resistance to spoiling. It is also great for cooking.

Buying and storing olive oil

When buying olive oil, check the 'sell-by' date; if the bottle also has a harvest date, avoid it if it is more than one year old. Also, avoid any bottle with a cork, as this can let air in and encourage oxidation.

Ideally, buy oil in an opaque container made from tin, ceramic or dark plastic. This is because light oxidizes the oil, lowering its levels of tocopherols (vitamin E), polyphenols and other antioxidants.

A study in Italy found that olive oil in a colourless bottle under supermarket lighting loses 30 per cent of its toco-pherols and carotenoids (which the body makes into vitamin A) over 12 months. After 2 months, the levels of peroxides (indicating the degree of oxidation and lowering of antioxidant levels) were so high that the oil could no longer be classed as extra virgin.

(*European Food Research and Technology*, 2005)

Brown or green glass bottles are second best but are usually the only containers available in supermarkets. Avoid buying a bottle that has been displayed in a shop window or under very bright lighting. At home, store olive oil in a dark place. You might enjoy looking at a beautiful bottle of olive oil, but it is better to keep the antioxidants intact.

Contact with air also uses up the antioxidants in virgin olive oil, so keep the container stoppered.

Exposure to heat can use up antioxidants, too, so store your olive oil in a cool place. You could transfer some oil from a big bottle to a small one, then store the big one in the refrigerator and keep the other at room temperature so it is ready to use. Refrigerated olive oil goes cloudy and thick and may even solidify, as olive oil needs a temperature of 40°F (4.4°C) or more to remain liquid. At 35°F (1.7°C) most olive oils are too thick to pour. As the temperature falls, first the heavier oils and waxes crystallize, then the lighter ones. Olive oil hardens in the freezer. However, neither refrigerating nor freezing does any harm, and the oil regains its normal appearance and consistency when restored to room temperature. Don't be dismayed if olive oil is cloudy at room temperature: this is often caused by microscopic fragments of olives. Some olive-oil processors 'winterize' their oil by removing its waxes so it remains clear when stored in a refrigerator.

The longer olive oil is around, the more it is exposed to light, air and heat, so:

- Use it within one month of opening the bottle.

- Consider buying a smaller bottle that you will use up more quickly.

- Buy olive oil only from a shop with a high turnover.

- Make olive oil your only added fat, so that you use it up quickly.

Researchers in Spain found that the content of chlorophyll, carotenoids and phenols dropped dramatically when virgin olive oil was stored for 12 months even in excellent conditions. Chlorophyll fell by 30 per cent, beta carotene (which the body can make into vitamin A) by 40 per cent, and alpha tocopherol (vitamin E) by 100 per cent; the polyphenols fell considerably too.

(*Journal of Agriculture and Food Chemistry*, 2007)

Cooking with olive oil

Extra virgin and virgin olive oils are the most stable of all the common unrefined cooking oils when heated. In addition, they are more nutritious and rich in antioxidants – some of which will remain in the fried food – than are refined olive oil or other refined vegetable oils. So they provide the best fat for frying, roasting or baking.

The benefits of olive oil's high smoke point

Do not allow olive oil to smoke, as this would indicate burning, which means it is beginning to break down and will taste unpleasant. Also, smoke covers everything in a tenacious brown film. The International Olive Council (IOC) says that extra virgin olive oil smokes at around

SMOKE POINTS OF UNREFINED VEGETABLE OILS

Oil	°C	°F
Extra virgin olive	210	410
Coconut	177	350
Sesame	177	350
Corn (maize)	160	320
Peanut	160	320
Soybean	160	320
Walnut	160	320
Sunflower	107	225
Safflower	107	225

210°C (410°F). The better quality the oil, the lower its acidity and the higher its smoke point. Also, the less cloudy it is, the higher its smoke point. Extra virgin olive oil has a far higher smoke point than other unrefined vegetable oils. Most of the vegetable oils other than olive oil that are sold in supermarkets are refined. While any oil has a higher smoke point if it is refined, such oil has almost no flavour and a much lower polyphenol content than does its unrefined counterpart.

Extra virgin olive oil also has a higher smoke point than that of butter, which is 177°C (350°F), and of lard, which is 188°C (370°F).

Olive oil should not be mixed with other fats or vegetable oils for frying, as these have lower smoke points.

The more an oil is overheated past its smoke point, the nearer it comes to its 'flash point', meaning the temperature at which its decomposition products spontaneously ignite.

Food scientists say that extra virgin olive oil heated to 180°C (350°F) undergoes a little oxidation but retains most of its nutrients, polyphenols and other health-giving constituents. This temperature is plenty hot enough for deep-frying. The International Olive Council says olive oil can be reused four or five times for frying. However, be especially careful not to overheat pre-used olive oil, because repeated heating lowers its smoke point. If you reuse olive oil, strain out any remnants of cooked food by passing the oil through a paper coffee filter or a piece of muslin, then refrigerate it.

Frying is most successful in very hot oil, as this caramelizes the natural sugars in food, making it taste good. Also, such heat alters proteins in the food's surface, forming a crust which prevents the inside of the food soaking up oil, enabling it to cook by steaming in its own intrinsic water. So the challenge is to heat olive oil until it is hot enough for successful frying but not so hot that it smokes.

Experience teaches us how to fry food in oil without burning the oil or the food. A novice soon learns to shallow-fry, but when learning to deep-fry it can help to measure the oil temperature with a food thermometer. Some deep-fat fryers have one built-in; with others you can clip one to the pan.

When deep-frying, the oil should be at least 2in/5cm deep and the pieces of food added one by one – not all together, as this would lower the temperature of the oil too much.

Maintaining nutrient levels

Extra virgin olive oil is the winner when it comes to maintaining the nutrient level of fried food, as the study below illustrates.

Spanish researchers report that stir-frying broccoli reduced its levels of vitamin C and polyphenols more than those of

TEMPERATURES NEEDED FOR FRYING

Type of food being fried	Ideal temperature range of oil
Foods with a high water content, such as vegetables, potatoes or fruit	Medium: 130–145°C (266–293°F)
Foods coated in flour, bread-crumbs or batter	Hot: 155–170°C (311–338°F)
Small pieces of quickly fried foods, such as sardines or scallops	Very hot: 175–190°C (347–374°F)

its minerals. When they compared different oils (extra virgin olive oil, refined olive oil, and sunflower, peanut, soyabean and safflower oils) for stir-frying different samples of broccoli, only extra virgin olive oil, soybean oil, peanut oil and safflower oil enabled broccoli to retain its levels of glucosinolates (cancer-preventing substances). And only extra virgin olive oil and sunflower oil enabled broccoli to retain its level of vitamin C.

(*Journal of Food Science*, 2007)

Oxidation and hydrogenation

Olive oil's high proportion of monounsaturated fat means it suffers less than other common vegetable oils from oxidation by heat. Indeed, the amount of oxidation is low enough to be of no concern.

As for hydrogenation, this is an industrial process that is used to harden polyunsaturated fats, and it simply cannot happen with home cooking. Only small degrees of hydrogenation occur even when frying in a commercial kitchen (such as in a fast-food shop) with oil that has repeatedly been heated to very high temperatures. For the fact is that efficient hydrogenation requires hydrogen to be bubbled through a vegetable oil while it is heated for several hours in the presence of a catalyst.

Trans fats

Home cooking won't produce trans fats in olive oil or any other vegetable oil.

Using olive oil in other ways

Olive oil can also be used around the house, and even as a shaving cream.

Olive oil lamps

These have been used for millennia. They provide a lovely soft light with no smoke or smell and are available for purchase on the internet. For instructions on how to make one, see http://www.motherearth-news.com/Do-It-Yourself/Make-Olive-Oil-Lamp.aspx.

Olive oil polish

A polish for furniture, tiles, wooden floors and other hard surfaces can be made by mixing one part of olive oil to one part of vinegar. Apply this mixture, then burnish with a soft cloth.

Olive oil shaving cream

This is made by mixing extra virgin olive oil with an equal amount of liquid soap. The mixture is then applied to the skin. Not only does it make the skin suitably slippery and ready for the razor but the oil also has antibacterial and soothing qualities.

CHAPTER 7

Recipes

Please note:

- Each recipe serves 4.

- 1 tsp (teaspoon) = 5ml; 1 tbsp (tablespoon) = 15ml; 1 cup = 240ml/8fl oz

- All fruit and vegetables are medium-sized unless otherwise stated.

- All eggs are medium (US large) unless otherwise stated.

- If using a fan oven, reduce the temperature recommended in the recipe by 20°C/25°F.

- Please note that salt is included only when needed to cure or soften other ingredients or to enhance their flavour. Anyone who wants to can add salt at the table.

Extra virgin olive oil has a subtle, complex and delicious flavour that makes even the simplest of dishes into something special. People in olive-growing areas use olive oil as those in dairying cultures use butter: for example, instead of putting butter on their bread, they dip their bread into olive oil. They enjoy the oil just as it comes, adding only a little sea salt or black pepper, or maybe a shake of balsamic vinegar.

Flavourful extra virgin olive oil makes an excellent dressing sprinkled fresh on to salads, cooked vegetables and pizza. It's also great for mixing into cooked grains, such as couscous, tabbouleh and polenta. Lastly, extra virgin olive oil is an ingredient of many popular recipes for fish and meat, desserts and puddings. You can also make excellent biscuits (cookies and crackers), cakes and pastry with extra virgin olive oil. Some people prefer the less pronounced flavour of what is classified as 'olive oil' (extra virgin oil mixed with refined oil) for certain dishes, or choose to cut costs by using this instead of extra virgin olive oil.

If swapping olive oil for butter in a recipe, use 3 tbsp olive oil for every 50g/2oz/4 tbsp butter.

Starters And Salads

Olive oil is invaluable for salads and starters. Besides the recipes below, you might also like to make croutons. These cubes of one- or two-day-old bread, gently fried for 2–3 minutes in extra virgin olive oil until golden-brown, make a very moreish garnish for salads and soups.

OLIVE OIL MARINATED GOAT'S CHEESE ON GARLICKY TOAST

Goat's cheese marinated in extra virgin olive oil infused with herbs and honey is amazingly good when toasted on top of garlicky toasted bread (crostini). Whilst all toasted cheese (including Welsh rarebit) is delicious, this Italian version is fit for a party.

8oz/225g fresh soft goat's cheese

For the marinade:
3 tbsp balsamic vinegar
2 garlic cloves, crushed
1 tsp ground black pepper
10 cured green olives, pitted and chopped
2 tbsp fresh basil leaves or 1 tbsp dried
150ml/5fl oz/scant 2/3 cup extra virgin olive oil (plus more if
    necessary)

For the crostini:
8 slices of French bread
4 tbsp extra virgin olive oil
2 garlic cloves, crushed

To marinate the cheese, slice it into ¾in/2cm thick slices and put these into a wide-necked jar or a pudding basin.

Put the balsamic vinegar, garlic, pepper, olives, basil and olive oil into a bowl and mix well with a fork or whisk. Pour this marinade over the sliced cheese. If necessary, add more oil and turn the jar upside down and back to ensure the marinade covers the cheese and the flavourings are well mixed. Refrigerate for a week, turning the jar each day.

To make the crostini, preheat the oven to 180ºC/350ºF/gas 4. At the same time, remove the marinated cheese from the refrigerator.

Put the slices of bread on to a baking tray, brush them with the olive oil, then bake for 10 minutes or until crisp and golden. Remove them from the oven (leaving the oven on) and rub garlic over each one.

Put a slice of cheese on each crostino, then put the tray of cheese-topped crostini into the oven and bake until the cheese is golden and bubbling.

Serve the crostini warm, either just as they are or with a green salad.

CAPER, OLIVE AND ANCHOVY DIP (TAPENADE)

Tapéna is the Provencal word for capers – the flower-buds of the *Capparis spinosa* bush, which grows around the Mediterranean and in parts of Asia. The buds are hand picked, then cured in vinegar, wine or brine. Combining them with anchovies, olives and extra virgin olive oil makes a delectably piquant dip.

4oz/100g/heaped ¾ cup pitted black olives
3 tbsp drained capers
3oz/75g tinned anchovy fillets, drained
1 tsp Dijon mustard
1 garlic clove
ground black pepper
1 tsp fresh or ½ tsp dried thyme
4fl oz/120ml/½ cup extra virgin olive oil
juice and finely grated zest of 1 lemon

Put the olives, capers, anchovies, mustard, garlic, a good grinding of black pepper and thyme into a blender and whizz to a smooth paste. Slowly add the olive oil and lemon juice and zest, whizzing all the time. Serve with bread, crackers or crudités, or as an accompaniment to cold meat, fish or hard-boiled (hard-cooked) eggs.

CURED SARDINES IN EXTRA VIRGIN OLIVE OIL

Sardines prepared this way are similar to the boquerones (cured anchovies in oil) often served in Spain and Morocco with other light dishes or tapas.

Curing sardines in vinegar means you don't have to cook them; it also softens any tiny bones that may remain. Cured sardines covered in extra virgin olive oil keep in the refrigerator for at least 1 week.

12 fresh sardines
600ml/20fl oz/2½ cups white wine vinegar
ground black pepper
2 garlic cloves, crushed
small handful of parsley, chopped
450ml/16fl oz/scant 2 cups extra virgin olive oil

Use sharp kitchen scissors to top and tail the sardines and remove the fins. Slit each belly and discard the innards. Remove the backbone of each fish from inside (starting at the tail end), then rinse the filleted fish well.

Place the sardine fillets in a shallow dish, sprinkle with the vinegar and a good grinding of black pepper and refrigerate for 2–12 hours.

Sieve the sardine fillets to drain away the vinegar, then rinse with cold running water. Add the garlic, parsley and extra virgin olive oil, toss lightly and leave to marinate for at least 2 hours.

HUMMUS

Hummus is Arabic for chickpeas. The combination of ground cooked chickpeas and ground sesame seeds (tahini) is particularly good.

Using pre-cooked canned chickpeas, as below, is easier than using dried chickpeas. But if you do use the dried version, soak 4oz/100g/ ½ cup overnight in water containing ½ teaspoon of bicarbonate of soda (baking soda). Drain and rinse, then add double their volume of water plus ½ teaspoon bicarbonate of soda and boil for 3 hours, topping up with water as necessary. Reserve 2 tablespoons of the cooking liquid to use instead of liquid from the can, as below.

Hummus keeps in the refrigerator for up to 3 days and in the freezer for up to 1 month.

425g/15oz canned chickpeas, drained (2 tbsp liquid reserved)
1 tbsp tahini
1 tbsp lemon juice
2 garlic cloves, crushed
½ tsp ground cumin
pinch of paprika, plus extra to garnish
3 tbsp extra virgin olive oil
pitta bread or tortilla chips, to serve

Reserve a few whole chickpeas and place the rest with the reserved liquid in a blender with the tahini, lemon juice, garlic, cumin, paprika and olive oil. Whizz on low for 3 minutes until smooth. If necessary, add water until the consistency of the hummus resembles that of thick mayonnaise.

Put the hummus into a serving dish and garnish with the reserved whole chickpeas and a sprinkle of paprika. Serve with warm pitta bread or tortilla crisps as a starter or a side dish.

Alternative garnishes include:

- 1 small handful of parsley or coriander (cilantro) leaves

- 2 tbsp caramelized onions, roasted red bell peppers or chopped raw onion

- quartered hard-boiled eggs

- 2 tbsp *ful medames* (see recipe on page 103).

MUSHROOM SALAD

The firm consistency of freshly picked mushrooms makes them a perfect salad ingredient. Choose between ordinary field mushrooms or more unusual varieties, such as oyster or shiitake. The other ingredients of this salad must be of high quality, too, so select good country bread, fresh parsley and a fine-tasting extra virgin olive oil.

    2 garlic cloves, crushed
    4 slices of wholemeal bread, toasted on both sides
    120ml/4fl oz/½ cup extra virgin olive oil
    325g/12oz mushrooms, thinly sliced
    juice of 1 lemon
    ground black pepper
    small handful of fresh parsley, chopped
    50g/2oz Parmesan or pecorino cheese

Rub the garlic into each side of each piece of bread. Tear the bread into pieces 1–2in/2–5cm long and put them into a serving dish.

Pour 4 tablespoons of the olive oil over the bread, then stir in the mushrooms, lemon juice, a good grinding of black pepper to taste, parsley and remaining oil.

Use a potato peeler to make cheese shavings, then sprinkle these over the salad and serve at once.

JEWELLED WHEAT SALAD (TABBOULEH)

Wheat that has been soaked, cooked and cracked is called *bulgur* in Arabic. It is available in many larger supermarkets as well as Greek and Middle-Eastern groceries. To make bulgur, wheat grains are soaked in water to soften them slightly; this boosts their nutritional value by activating seed-growth enzymes. The grains are then boiled, dried, ground and graded.

Bulgur has a nutty flavour, and adding lemon juice, herbs and vegetables makes it into tabbouleh – the flavourful and colourful wheat salad that is the national dish of Lebanon.

100g/4oz/heaped ¾ cup fine bulgur
juice of 1 lemon
120ml/4fl oz/½ cup extra virgin olive oil
ground black pepper
1 onion, finely chopped
2 garlic cloves, peeled and crushed
3 tomatoes, chopped
2 handfuls of flat-leaf parsley, coarsely chopped
1 handful of mint, coarsely chopped
pitta bread and crisp lettuce leaves, to serve

Put the bulgur into a bowl, cover with 600ml/20fl oz/2½ cups boiling water and leave for 30 minutes to soften and expand.

Drain the bulgur in a sieve and press it with a tablespoon or your fingers to squeeze out the water. Stir in the lemon juice, olive oil and a good grinding of black pepper. Now stir in the onion, garlic, tomatoes, parsley and mint and place in the refrigerator for 30 minutes.

Serve as a starter with pitta bread and lettuce.

Salad Dressings, Sauces And Flavoured Oils

A good dressing made with extra virgin olive oil turns a salad of lettuce, rocket, chicory, chickweed or young dandelion leaves into a delight. Another idea is to dip raw vegetables, such as carrots, celery and radishes, into pinzinmonio – extra virgin olive oil flavoured with salt and a good grinding of black pepper.

The better quality the oil, the better the dressing. And just as you can enjoy discovering different wines, including single-estate wines, so too is it enjoyable to try different olive oils, including single-estate oils.

FRENCH DRESSING (VINAIGRETTE)

Whatever you decide to put into your French dressing (see the suggested additions below), ensure that all the ingredients are at room temperature when you begin. This is because the colder they are, the more difficult it is to combine them into a smooth emulsion.

    120ml/4fl oz/½ cup extra virgin olive oil
    2 tbsp apple cider vinegar or white wine vinegar
    1 tsp Dijon mustard
    1 tsp clear honey
    1 garlic clove, crushed
    salt and ground black pepper

Either put all the ingredients into a bowl, season with a pinch of salt and a good grinding of black pepper, then whisk well with a fork *or* put them into a screw-top container, screw on the lid and shake the container well. Pour the dressing over the salad leaves just before serving, and toss the leaves to coat them in the dressing.

You can keep the dressing at room temperature for up to 3 hours; if it separates out, simply shake it or mix it with a fork again before it's needed. Alternatively, keep it in the refrigerator for a week, removing it 2 hours before wanted, and shake it or mix it with a fork to emulsify it just before serving.

Variations

- substitute some of the extra virgin olive oil with walnut or hazelnut oil

- substitute some or all of the white wine vinegar with another vinegar (such as balsamic or tarragon) or lemon (or other citrus) juice

- add less oil and more vinegar

- add more or less mustard and more or less honey

- add 1 tbsp chopped fresh herbs (such as basil) or 1 tsp dried herbs

- add 1 tsp celery seed

- add ½ tsp paprika

- stir in 2 tsp mayonnaise.

MAYONNAISE

A blender allows you to prepare this lovely mayonnaise quickly and without fear of it curdling. Using a hand whisk is just as successful but takes a little longer.

> 1 egg
> 1 tsp Dijon mustard
> ½ tsp caster (superfine) sugar
> 300ml/10½fl oz/1¼ cups extra virgin olive oil
> ground black pepper
> 2 tsp wine vinegar

Put the egg, mustard, sugar, 4 tablespoons of the olive oil and a good grinding of black pepper into a blender. Whizz until smooth. Uncover, then, with the blender at medium speed, slowly drizzle in 150ml/ 5fl oz/scant ⅔ cup of the oil, and then the vinegar. Whizz until the mixture is smooth, then slowly add the remaining oil. Whizz again until the mayonnaise is thick, then add 4 teaspoons boiling water and whizz slowly until well mixed.

Tip: If you are making the mayonnaise with a hand whisk and it curdles, remedy the problem by putting an egg yolk into another bowl, adding the curdled mayonnaise, then beating well.

Variations

- For lemon mayonnaise, substitute lemon juice for the wine vinegar and add 1 teaspoon finely grated lemon zest

- For herb mayonnaise, chop a handful of fresh herbs (such as basil, marjoram or chervil) and stir into the mayonnaise.

GARLICKY RED PEPPER SAUCE

This lovely garlicky sauce makes a terrific accompaniment for oily fish such as herring or tuna. It's also simply scrumptious when floated along with some croûtons on the top of a bowl of bouillabaisse (fish 'stew') or fish soup.

    1 red bell pepper
    2 slices of bread
    2 garlic cloves, peeled
    4 tbsp extra virgin olive oil
    1 tbsp fish stock

Put the red pepper on to a baking tray under a pre-heated grill (broiler) and grill (broil) it, turning it several times, until the skin becomes slightly charred. Remove it from the heat, allow to cool slightly, then remove the skin, seeds and thick pieces of pith.

Make the bread into breadcrumbs using a blender. Cover these with water, then drain in a sieve and squeeze out the extra water by hand.

Put the pepper, breadcrumbs, garlic, olive oil and fish stock into the blender and whizz until smooth.

Serve with fish, fish stew or fish soup.

FLAVOURED OLIVE OIL

Marinating herbs or spices in extra virgin olive oil transfers their aromatic flavours to the oil. Flavoured oils make excellent salad dressings and are good for cooking vegetables, fish, poultry and meat. They are also delectable as a dip for chunks of bread.

1 litre/35fl oz/4-cup bottle of extra virgin olive oil

1 tbsp lemon juice

One of these flavourings:

2 tbsp dried basil, chervil, coriander (cilantro), dill, marjoram, mint, oregano, parsley, sage or tarragon

5 dried bay leaves

2 tbsp black peppercorns, cumin or coriander seeds, cardamom pods or juniper berries

finely pared peel of 2 lemons, patted dry with kitchen paper

3 small dried red chillies

Pour 240ml/8fl oz/1 cup of the oil into a jug, to make room in the bottle for the flavouring, and keep this oil to one side. Stuff the chosen herb or spice into the bottle. Refill the bottle with as much of the reserved oil as possible, then put the top back on the bottle and refrigerate it.

Consume the flavoured oil within 1 month.

Vegetables

The marriage of vegetables and extra virgin olive oil is made in heaven. Anointing raw salad vegetables with this aromatic, slightly bitter oil (see 'Salad Dressings, Sauces and Flavoured Oils', page 96) makes them much more attractive to eat. This encourages us to eat more of them and thus benefit from their wealth of vitamins, minerals, plant pigments and salicylates. As for cooking vegetables with extra virgin olive oil, this not only adds to their flavour but also helps to preserve their texture and moistness.

The following recipes for cooking beans and pulses, Mediterranean vegetables, spinach and potatoes with extra virgin olive oil are excellent examples of dishes that are both health-giving and popular.

GARLICKY SPINACH WITH OLIVE OIL

Cooking spinach with extra virgin olive oil gives it an even more luscious texture than usual and also makes it taste utterly glorious!

1.3kg/3lb spinach, well washed
180ml/6fl oz/¾ cup extra virgin olive oil
3 garlic cloves, crushed
ground black pepper

Put the wet spinach into a large saucepan, cook gently until it wilts, then drain. Squeeze out as much as possible of the water remaining in the spinach, then finely chop it.

Put the extra virgin olive oil and garlic into a frying pan and fry the garlic gently for a minute. Add the spinach and cook it, stirring occasionally, until it absorbs all the oil. Stir in a good grinding of black pepper and serve hot as an accompanying vegetable, or with a poached egg as a light main course.

BROAD BEANS WITH LEMON AND GARLIC
(FUL MEDAMES)

This dish is made from broad beans – the seeds of the *Vicia faba* plant that are also known as fava, faba and horse beans. Ful medames is Egypt's national dish, 'ful' meaning fava beans and 'medames' meaning buried. Centuries ago, a pot of beans and water would have been buried in a fire and slow-cooked for hours.

If you are using fresh broad beans, note that around 1.3kg/3lb of broad bean pods yields about 450g/1lb actual beans.

450g/1lb/2½ cups fresh broad beans (450g/1lb/scant 3 cups
    frozen broad beans), cooked and drained, but with 240ml/8fl
    oz/1 cup of the cooking liquid reserved.
OR 750g/1lb/10oz canned broad beans, drained, but with
    240ml/8fl oz/1 cup of the liquid reserved
3 tbsp extra virgin olive oil
juice of 1 lemon
2 tsp ground cumin
4 garlic cloves, crushed
2 tbsp parsley, chopped

Put half the beans into a bowl with the reserved liquid, and mash with a potato masher. Stir in the remaining beans, olive oil, lemon juice, cumin and garlic.

Put this mixture into individual bowls, sprinkle with chopped parsley and serve with hard-boiled eggs and bread as a starter or a side dish. Alternatively, serve as a light main course with yoghurt or feta cheese and chopped tomatoes and onions.

AUBERGINES BAKED WITH TOMATOES, ONIONS AND CHEESE (MELANZANE PARMIGIANA)

This warming comfort food is easy to make at home and is also one of the most popular starters or vegetarian main courses in Italian restaurants. Some people deseed and skin the tomatoes, but I do this only if cooking for someone who prefers to avoid the skins and seeds, as I like their appearance, texture and nutritional value.

240ml/8fl oz/1 cup extra virgin olive oil

2 onions, chopped

3 garlic cloves, finely chopped

180ml/6fl oz/¾ cup red wine

small handful of fresh oregano, chopped, or 2 tsp dried oregano

800g/1¾lb fresh or canned tomatoes, coarsely chopped

ground black pepper

3 aubergines (eggplant), cut into ¾in/2cm slices

325g/12oz mozzarella cheese, cut into 1cm/½in slices

100g/4oz/1 cup grated Parmesan cheese

Heat 2 tablespoons of the olive oil in a heavy-based casserole, add the onions and garlic and fry gently for about 5 minutes to soften the onion. Add the wine and the dried oregano (if using fresh oregano, you add it later), and heat until bubbling, then simmer for another 5 minutes. Add the tomatoes and return to the boil, then simmer, stirring occasionally, for 30 minutes. If using fresh oregano, stir this in now. Meanwhile, preheat the oven to 200°C/400°F/gas 6.

Put the remaining oil and a good grinding of black pepper into a large bowl, add the aubergines and toss them well. Put a layer of aubergine slices into a large frying pan and fry them gently for about

3 minutes on each side. Put them on to a plate and repeat with the remaining aubergine slices.

Put half the tomato mixture into an oiled, heavy-based casserole, cover with half the aubergine slices, then with half the cheese. Repeat the layers.

Turn the oven down to 180°C/350°F/gas 4 and bake for 45 minutes, covering the top of the dish with aluminium foil if necessary to prevent excessive browning.

GOLDEN FRIED POTATOES

Potatoes fried in extra virgin olive oil have a wonderful flavour with a slight, but attractive, hint of bitterness.

> 4 medium–large potatoes, thickly sliced
> 1 tsp salt
> juice of 1 lemon
> 480ml/16fl oz/2 cups extra virgin olive oil

Put the potatoes into a large shallow pan, sprinkle with the salt and lemon juice and stir well. Cover and leave for 45 minutes.

Put the extra olive oil into a deep saucepan and heat it to 180–185°C/350–365°F. To know when the temperature is right, either use a food thermometer or drop a little cube of bread into the oil – if the oil is hot enough, the bread will immediately rise, sizzling, to the surface.

Add the potatoes and fry gently, stirring occasionally, until golden-brown.

Remove the potatoes and put them on a wire rack over kitchen paper to drain. Serve hot.

BAKED MEDITERRANEAN VEGETABLES (RATATOUILLE)

This medley of cooked tomatoes, courgettes (zucchini), aubergines (eggplant) and bell peppers (which in botanical terms are fruits rather than vegetables) is cooked with extra virgin olive oil and fragranced with garlic, thyme and basil. Enjoy it as a starter, an accompaniment to meat, fish, eggs or pasta, or in a quiche. Cooking the vegetables separately takes longer but keeps the flavours nicely distinct.

2 onions, sliced
150ml/5fl oz/scant ⅔ cup extra virgin olive oil
4 garlic cloves, finely chopped
2 aubergines, thickly sliced
3 courgettes, thickly sliced
2 red or yellow bell peppers, deseeded and quartered
4 ripe tomatoes, sliced
salt
black pepper
3 thyme sprigs
handful of basil leaves

Gently fry the onions in 2 tablespoons of the olive oil for 5 minutes or until soft. Add the garlic and continue to cook for a further minute. Put the mixture into a baking dish. Gently fry each of the other types of vegetable separately, each time adding 2 tablespoons of the oil, cooking for 5 minutes, then addding to the baking dish. Season with salt and a good grinding of black pepper, add the thyme leaves and stir gently.

Bake at 180°C/350°F/gas 4 for 45 minutes. Sprinkle with the basil leaves and serve.

TOMATO TART

Gently frying tomatoes in extra virgin olive oil or other fat makes their red plant pigment lycopene more easily absorbed by our digestive tract. Lycopene is an antioxidant and is believed to help counteract inflammation, allergy and, perhaps, certain cancers.

450g/1lb puff pastry
450g/1lb tomatoes, halved
120ml/4fl oz/½ cup extra virgin olive oil
2 garlic cloves, finely chopped
2 tsp sugar
12 tomatoes, finely sliced
small handful of basil leaves, chopped

Preheat the oven to 220°C/425°F/gas mark 7.

Roll the pastry into a 30cm/12in circle, place on a greased baking sheet and put in the refrigerator for 30 minutes.

Put the halved tomatoes, 3 tablespoons of the olive oil, the garlic and sugar in a saucepan and cook gently for 10 minutes. Remove from the heat, tip into a blender and whizz for 1 minute or until it has the consistency of a thick sauce. Leave to cool for 5 minutes.

Spread the tomato sauce over the pastry circle, leaving a small (1cm/½in) border bare all around. Arrange the sliced tomatoes on top and sprinkle with another 3 tablespoons of the olive oil.

Turn the oven down to 180°C/350°F/gas 4 and bake the tart for about 30 minutes, or until the tomatoes are slightly browned but not burning.

Remove from the oven, sprinkle with the remaining olive oil and the basil, and serve hot or cold.

Pasta and Pizza

Extra virgin olive oil is an ingredient of many traditional Italian recipes, including pasta dishes and pizzas. Not only is extra virgin olive oil included in traditional pasta sauces but it is also a basic ingredient of pizza dough. And in Italy and in Italian restaurants olive oil is often sprinkled liberally over a pizza immediately after it has been cooked.

PASTA WITH EXTRA VIRGIN OLIVE OIL AND GARLIC (AGLIO E OLIO)

One way of preparing this Italian favourite is simply to splash freshly cooked spaghetti or other pasta with extra virgin olive oil and stir in half a dozen cloves of freshly crushed garlic and a good grinding of black pepper. If you would like a little more guidance, follow the recipe below.

> 180ml/6fl oz/¾ cup extra virgin olive oil
> 6 garlic cloves, crushed
> handful of basil or parsley, chopped
> ground black pepper
> 120ml/4fl oz/½ cup white wine
> 550g/1¼lb pasta, cooked al dente

Into a large saucepan put the olive oil, garlic, basil or parsley, a good grinding of black pepper and white wine. Bring to the boil and simmer for 3–4 minutes, stirring constantly. Pour this sauce over the pasta, stir gently and serve.

PIZZA MARGHERITA

When Queen Margherita visited the Palace of Capodimonte in Naples in 1889, she asked eminent chef Raffaele Esposito to cook pizza. He made pizza mastunicola (with cheese, lard and basil), pizza marinara (tomatoes, garlic, oil and oregano) ... and a pizza with the colours of the Italian flag – red, white and green from tomatoes, mozzarella and basil – but no name. This last one was her favourite, so the chef named it pizza margherita.

225g/8oz/2 cups wholemeal bread flour
225g/8oz/1½ cups white bread flour
1 x 7g/¼oz sachet of dried (dry active) yeast
1 tsp salt
1 tbsp caster (superfine) sugar
6 tbsp extra virgin olive oil
350g/12oz tomatoes
300g/1⅓oz mozzarella, thinly sliced
small handful of basil leaves

Put the flours, yeast, salt and sugar into a large bowl and make a well in the centre. Pour half the olive oil and 330ml/11fl oz/1⅓ cups tepid water into the well and mix into the dry ingredients. Knead thoroughly by hand or with the dough hook of a food mixer for 10 minutes. Cover with a damp cloth and leave to rise in a warm place for at least 2 hours or until doubled in size.

Roll the dough into a circle about 6mm/¼in thick, transfer to a baking tray and prick all over with a fork.

Crush the tomatoes with a fork and spread over the pizza base. Leave to rise a little for 30 minutes in a warm place. Meanwhile, preheat the oven to 240°C/475°F/gas 9.

Turn the oven down to 200°C/400°F/gas 6. Put the pizza into the oven and cook for 20 minutes.

Remove from the oven, place the mozzarella slices on top and sprinkle with the remaining oil and the basil. Return the pizza to the oven and cook for 10 minutes. Remove and serve hot.

PASTA PESTO

This lovely pasta sauce is quick and easy to make. The word 'pesto' comes from the Italian *pestare*, meaning 'to pound'. You can vary the ingredients by substituting walnuts, cashew nuts or hazelnuts for the pine nuts; rocket or flat-leaf parsley for the basil; and/or pecorino cheese for the Parmesan.

2 large handfuls of basil leaves
150ml/¼ pint/⅔ cup extra virgin olive oil
2 garlic cloves
100g/3½oz/⅔ cup pine nuts
50g/2oz Parmesan, cut into small pieces
freshly cooked pasta, to serve

Put all the ingredients apart from the pasta into a blender and whizz until well blended.

Stir this pesto into the pasta and serve at once. Alternatively, put it into a covered container and refrigerate for up to 1 week.

Eggs, Poultry, Meat, Fish

Olive oil is a good oil to use when frying, grilling or roasting because it adds flavour and, unlike many other vegetable oils, it isn't damaged at the temperatures generally used for home cooking. A herb- or spice-flavoured olive oil also makes an excellent marinade for meat, poultry or fish.

FISH WITH TOMATO AND OLIVE OIL SAUCE

Whether the fish is white or oily makes no difference because any fish is good with this delicious sauce. You can use either filleted fish or fish on the bone.

240ml/8fl oz/1 cup extra virgin olive oil
4 tomatoes, chopped
ground black pepper
juice and zest of 1 lemon
900g/2lb plaice, herring or other fish
small handful of dill, snipped

Put the olive oil, tomatoes and a good grinding of black pepper into a pan and fry gently, stirring occasionally, for 3–5 minutes, until the tomatoes are soft but not brown. Stir in the lemon juice and zest. Turn off the heat and leave the sauce in the pan.

Fry, bake, grill (broil) or microwave the fish, taking care not to overcook it.

Re-heat the tomato and olive oil sauce, if necessary, then pour over the fish. Sprinkle with the dill and serve immediately.

EGGS WITH PEPPERS, ONIONS AND TOMATOES (PIPERADE)

The name piperade comes from the Latin word 'piper', meaning pepper, and many older recipes contained both bell peppers and chilli peppers. A typical recipe today contains only mild peppers along with onions, tomatoes and, of course, extra virgin olive oil. The Spanish omelette is a popular spin-off of such recipes.

4 tbsp extra virgin olive oil

1 red onion, finely sliced

2 garlic cloves, finely chopped

2 green bell peppers, deseeded and finely sliced

1 red bell pepper, deseeded and finely sliced

2 tomatoes, coarsely chopped

ground black pepper

4 eggs, beaten

small handful of basil leaves, roughly torn

4 slices of good fresh bread

Put 3 tablespoons of the olive oil and the onion into a large frying pan. Fry gently for 5 minutes or until the onion begins to soften. Add the garlic and green and red peppers and cook for 8–10 minutes. Stir in the tomatoes and a good grinding of black pepper and cook for 3 minutes.

Heat the remaining oil in a small non-stick pan, add the eggs and cook, stirring, for 2–3 minutes or until the eggs are just set. Stir the scrambled eggs into the pan of peppers and tomatoes.

Spoon the mixture on to the bread and sprinkle it with fresh basil.

CHICKEN WITH OLIVES

Use chicken thighs with or without their skin for this recipe, according to your personal taste. Alternatively, substitute four chicken quarters or breasts for the thighs. Whatever you choose, the result will be fragrant and full of flavour.

8 chicken thighs
180ml/6fl oz/¾ cup extra virgin olive oil
2 green bell peppers, deseeded and sliced
2 red bell peppers, deseeded and sliced
2 onions, sliced
2 garlic cloves, finely chopped
225g/8oz/scant 2 cups pitted black olives
3 tomatoes, finely sliced
240ml/8fl oz/1 cup red wine
good bread or mashed potatoes, to serve

Preheat the oven to 180ºC/350ºF/gas 4.

Put the chicken thighs and olive oil into a heavy-based casserole. Add the remaining ingredients.

Cover the casserole, put it into the oven and cook for 1½ hours, turning the chicken thighs half-way through the cooking time. Serve hot with good bread, or with potatoes.

PORK WITH SAGE AND GARLIC

There will be a wonderfully appetising aroma in your kitchen if you cook pork in extra virgin olive oil in which you have gently fried sage and bay leaves and black pepper. And when you eat the pork, its flavour will certainly not disappoint!

6 tbsp extra virgin olive oil
2 garlic cloves, finely chopped
small handful of sage leaves, coarsely chopped
ground black pepper
4 bay leaves
675g/1½lb lean leg of pork, cut into 2.5cm/1in cubes
180ml/6fl oz/¾ cup white wine
mashed potatoes and a green vegetable, to serve

Heat the olive oil in a frying pan and add the garlic, sage, a good grinding of black pepper and bay leaves. Fry gently for 2–3 minutes, being sure not to burn the garlic or sage. Add the pork and fry, turning frequently, for 5 minutes. Add half the wine and cook, turning occasionally, for 10 minutes.

Put the pork on to hot plates. Add the remaining wine to the pan and heat for 1 minute, stirring well. Pour the pan juices over the pork and serve with mashed potatoes and a green vegetable.

BEEF KEBABS

Soaking beef and vegetables in an olive oil-rich marinade adds to their flavour and succulence. For a change, try substituting pork or chicken for the beef, and chunks of bell pepper and aubergine (eggplant) for the courgette (zucchini) and tomatoes.

240ml/8fl oz/1 cup extra virgin olive oil

3 tbsp cider vinegar

3 garlic cloves, crushed

small handful of parsley, chopped

ground black pepper

550g/1¼lb sirloin or top round beef, cut into 2.5cm/1in cubes
and with any visible fat removed

1 courgette (zucchini), cut into 1cm/½in slices

12 small tomatoes

Put the olive oil, cider vinegar, garlic, parsley and a good grinding of black pepper into a bowl and stir well. Add the beef, courgette and tomatoes and stir. Leave for 2 hours at room temperature or overnight in the refrigerator.

Use a slotted spoon to drain and transfer the beef, courgettes and tomatoes to a large plate, reserving the marinade.

Thread the beef, courgettes and tomatoes on to long steel kebab skewers, ending each one with a cube of beef.

Put the kebabs on to an oiled baking sheet and brush them with the marinade. Heat the grill (broiler).

Put the kebabs under the grill, 10cm/4in from the flames, and cook for 3 minutes for medium-rare beef or 4–5 minutes for medium–well-done. Turn the kebabs over, brush with more marinade and cook for the same time again.

Biscuits, Cakes, Desserts, Pastry and Breads

Extra virgin olive oil is a brilliant fat to use when baking cakes and biscuits and for making puddings and other desserts. It produces a lovely smooth texture and infuses food with its subtly bitter and aromatic flavour.

Traditional recipes of non-dairying countries have often used extra virgin olive oil or some other kind of vegetable oil for baking breads, biscuits, cakes and desserts. People in dairying countries are more familiar with the use of butter, margarine or other solid fats (such as lard, used as in lardy cake in the UK). But it is interesting to experiment by swapping the solid fat that you usually use for extra virgin olive oil.

Don't forget, too, that you can mix and match different oils. For example, if a recipe suggests using 120ml/4fl oz/½ cup of extra virgin olive oil, but you think a slightly nutty flavour would be even better, simply substitute walnut or hazelnut oil for half the volume of the olive oil.

SESAME BISCUITS

Making biscuits (crackers) with olive oil means they keep longer than other biscuits. Their texture is wonderfully crumbly and a little drier than that of most other biscuits.

100g/4oz/³⁄₄ cup sesame seeds

360ml/12fl oz/1½ cups olive oil

juice and finely grated zest of ½ lemon

3 tbsp brandy

1 tsp cinnamon

1 tsp ground cloves

150g/5oz/²⁄₃ cup caster (superfine) sugar

400g/14oz/3¼ cups self-raising (self-rising) flour, sifted

Put the sesame seeds into a very fine sieve, wash under cold, running water and leave to drain for 1 hour.

Put the olive oil, lemon juice and zest, brandy, cinnamon, cloves and 6 tbsp hot water into another bowl and beat well. Add the sugar and beat for about 5 minutes. Stir in the flour, then knead for 10 minutes, adding more flour if necessary to prevent the dough sticking to your hands.

Preheat the oven to 220°C/425°F/gas 7.

Take a walnut-sized piece of dough and shape it into an oval, round, ring, plait, spiral, figure of eight or twist. Dip this into the sesame seeds and push them in to secure them. Put the sesame-coated shapes on a nonstick or greased baking sheet, leaving gaps between them. Repeat until you have used all the dough.

Reduce the heat to 180°C/350°C/gas 4 and cook for 15–20 minutes or until the biscuits are light brown. Leave the biscuits to cool on the baking sheet, then serve at once. Alternatively, because they contain no butter or eggs, you can store them in an airtight container at room temperature for up to 2 months, or freeze them for up to about 3 months.

ROCK CAKES

My mother used to make rock cakes, and as a child I always loved the enticing aroma that wafted from the oven as they baked. This recipe is similar to hers, but contains extra virgin olive oil instead of butter.

5 tbsp extra virgin olive oil

75g/3oz/scant ½ cup golden caster (unrefined superfine) sugar

1 egg, beaten

100g/4oz/¾ cup sultanas (golden raisins)

grated zest of 1 orange

225g/8oz/1¾ cups self-raising (self-rising) flour

pinch of mixed (apple pie) spice

Preheat the oven to 180ºC/350ºC/gas 4

Put all the ingredients into a large bowl and stir well. Put 10–12 spoonfuls of the dough on to a greased baking tray spaced a little apart and bake for 15–20 minutes. Leave to cool on the tray.

SAVOURY OLIVE OIL BISCUITS

These biscuits (crackers) have a delightfully unusual texture and go well with soup and many other starters, or with cheese. You can vary their flavour by adding either grated Parmesan or dried herbs to the dough.

250g/9oz/2 cups self-raising (self-rising) flour, sifted
1 tsp ground black pepper
5 tbsp extra virgin olive oil
185ml/6fl oz/¾ cup milk, buttermilk or plain full-fat yoghurt
Optional: 75g/3oz/¾ cup grated Parmesan or 2 tsp dried
   oregano leaves

Preheat the oven to 220°C/425°F/gas 7.

Put the flour in a bowl and stir in the black pepper. Put the olive oil and 170ml/5½fl oz/⅔ cup of the buttermilk into another bowl and stir well. Make a well in the flour mixture, add the olive-oil mixture and stir thoroughly. Add the remaining milk and stir again.

Put the dough on to a lightly floured work surface and use your hands to press it out to 1cm/½in thick, then fold it in half. Repeat the pressing and folding five times, then press out again. Stamp out rounds with a cookie cutter and place on a greased baking sheet.

Reduce the oven temperature to 180°C/350°F/gas 4. Bake the biscuits for about 10 minutes until they are golden brown. Transfer to a wire rack to cool.

OLIVE OIL SPONGE CAKE

Butter may be the most popular fat for cake-making in the US, Australia and Western Europe, but it certainly isn't the only one, let alone the best one, for this purpose. In many countries other fats, or vegetable oils such as olive oil, are used with great success.

This sponge cake, made with olive oil, is very enjoyable when served just as it is but is also good when frosted with a glacé or butter-icing topping.

> 5 eggs
> 150g/5oz/¾ cup golden caster (unrefined superfine) sugar
> 2 tbsp extra virgin olive oil
> 150g/5oz/1¼ cups plain (all-purpose) flour
> 2 tbsp icing (confectioner's) sugar

Preheat the oven to 170°C/325°F/gas 3.

Grease a 23cm/9in springform tin and put a circle of non-stick baking paper on its base.

Put the eggs into a bowl and whisk with an electric mixer for 3 minutes or until the mixture is pale and thick. Add the caster sugar and keep whisking until the mixture leaves a trail when you lift out the beaters. Continue to whisk at high speed while very slowly adding the olive oil. Sift the flour on to the mixture and fold in with a spoon.

Pour into the tin and bake for 40–45 minutes until the cake is golden and springy and shrinking away from the sides of the tin. Leave to cool for 10 minutes in the tin, then turn out on to a wire rack. Sift the icing sugar over the top.

CARROT AND APPLE CAKE

This recipe makes a lovely moist cake that serves at least 12. You can increase the amount of cinnamon if you are particularly fond of it.

350g12oz/2¾ cups plain (all-purpose) flour
1 tbsp bicarbonate of soda (baking soda)
½ tsp cinnamon
½ tsp mace
1 tsp salt
2 eggs
4 egg whites
300ml/10½fl oz/1¼ cups extra virgin olive oil
350g/12oz/1½ cups caster (superfine) sugar
240ml/8fl oz/1 cup unsweetened stewed apple
2 tsp vanilla extract
675g/1½lb carrots, peeled and grated
150g/5oz/1 cup sultanas (golden raisins)
100g/4oz/¾ cup chopped walnuts
icing (confectioner's) sugar, to dust (optional)

Preheat the oven to 180°C/350°F/gas 4.

Grease a 23 x 33cm/9 x 13in cake tin and lightly dust with flour.

Sift the flour, bicarbonate of soda, cinnamon, mace and salt into a bowl and mix well.

Put the eggs, egg whites, olive oil, caster sugar, stewed apple and vanilla essence into a large bowl and beat with a wooden spoon until very well mixed. Stir in the grated carrots. Add the flour mixture and beat for 3 minutes. Stir in the sultanas and nuts.

Pour the mixture into the cake tin. Bake for 1 hour 15 minutes or until the cake shrinks away from the sides of the tin and an inserted metal skewer comes out clean. Put on a wire rack to cool.

Sprinkle with icing sugar, if wanted.

DELICIOUS YOGHURT PUDDING

This pudding has a melt-in-the-mouth texture and a citrus tang. It is delightful hot or cold and either on its own or with stewed or fresh fruit. Greek yoghurt adds creaminess, but full-fat plain yoghurt flavoured with coconut is a delicious alternative.

3 eggs, separated
120ml/4fl oz/½ cup extra virgin olive oil
100g/4oz/½ cup caster (superfine) sugar
finely grated zest of 1 lemon
300ml/10½fl oz/1¼ cups Greek yoghurt
75g/3oz/⅔ cup self-raising (self-rising) flour, sifted

Preheat the oven to 170°C/325°F/gas 3.

Put the egg whites into a bowl and whisk until stiff. Put the olive oil, sugar, egg yolks, lemon zest and yoghurt into another bowl, and whisk until well mixed. Stir in the flour, then fold in the beaten egg whites.

Pour the mixture into a greased baking dish and bake for 30 minutes. Serve warm with hot stewed apricots, apples, prunes or figs, or cold with fresh red grapes or mixed berries.

OLIVE OIL PASTRY

This recipe uses olive oil instead of butter or other fat and makes enough pastry dough to line a 28–30cm/11–12in tart tin. The finished pastry has an excellent texture and flavour.

> 250g/9oz/2 cups plain (all-purpose) flour (or half and half plain and wholemeal flours)
> *for a savoury recipe*: 1 tsp fine sea salt and 1 tsp dried mixed herbs
> *for a sweet recipe*: 2 tbsp caster (superfine) sugar
> 6 tbsp extra virgin olive oil

Put the flour and either the salt and dried herbs or the sugar into a bowl. Stir in the olive oil and most of 120ml/4fl oz/½ cup cold water. Work the dough with your hands until it forms a ball, adding the remaining water if necessary.

Put the dough into a bowl, cover with cling film (plastic wrap) and rest in the refrigerator for 30 minutes. Use as required within a day.

HERBY OLIVE BREAD

This aromatic bread is best served warm, perhaps with a glass of red wine or a bowl of tomato soup. As a variation, you could swap the olives for sun-dried tomatoes.

  1kg/2lb 4oz/8 cups white bread flour
  3 x 7g/¼oz sachets dried (dry active) yeast
  1 tbsp dried basil
  1 tbsp caster (superfine) sugar
  1 tsp salt
  5 tbsp extra virgin olive oil
  150g/5oz/1 cup pitted Kalamata olives, chopped
  butter, for greasing

Put the flour, yeast, basil, sugar, salt, olive oil, olives and 600ml/20fl oz/2½ cups warm water into a large bowl and stir well. Bring the dough together with your hands, then turn out on to a floured surface and knead for 5 minutes. Cover the bowl with cling film (plastic wrap) and leave in a warm room for about 45 minutes or until the dough has doubled in size.

Grease a baking tray. Knead the dough again for 1 minute then put it on the tray and shape it into a long, rounded loaf. Cover with a cloth and leave to rise for about 1 hour until doubled in size. Meanwhile, preheat the oven to 180°C/350°F/gas 4.

Bake for about 45 minutes until slightly browned on top. Leave the bread on the tray for 2 minutes or so, then remove and cool on a wire rack.

Useful addresses and websites

Many countries have shops devoted to olive oil and olive products and many olive-growing countries have festivals to celebrate the olive harvest. You can find information on the internet about these and about the many olive-oil producers around the world.

Here is a selection of other companies and organizations concerned with olive oil.

Italy
Experience the Olive Harvest
Tel: 0039 075 845457
www.rogaia.com

An olive farm that offers holidays to experience the olive harvest and enables you to adopt an olive tree and receive extra virgin olive oil from the farm.

Spain
International Olive Council (IOC)
Tel: 0034 91 590 36 38
www.internationaloliveoil.org

This trade organization, set up under the auspices of the United Nations, encourages international trade in olive oil and cooperation on research, development, technology and training. It also promotes consumption of olive oil, updates standards of olive oil quality, and supplies information on the world's market. Importantly, it represents the marketing of over 95 per cent of the world's olive-oil production and its quality standards for olive oil are used by many olive oil producing countries, including Spain, Italy, Greece, Portugal and Turkey. The IOC's standards are recognized by the vast majority of the world's olive-oil producers and marketers. The new standards in the US are largely based on those of the IOC.

United States
The United States Agriculture Department

Sets standards for olive oils marketed in the US: see http://www.ams.usda.gov/AMSv1.0/getfile?dDocName=STELDEV3011889

California Olive Oil Council
Tel: 001 888 718 9830
www.cooc.com

Provides news and other information about olive oil, promotes olive oil, and offers producers its Seal programme to certify that oils are what they are claimed to be.

Texas Olive Oil Council
Tel: 001 214 325 5787
www.texasoliveoilcouncil.org

Provides information about olive oil and promotes high standards for olive farming.

The Olive Oil Source
Tel: 001 805 688 1014
www.oliveoilsource.com

Provides information about olive oil and sells olive oil and products made from olive oil.

Australia
Australian Olive Oil Association
Tel: 0061 3 9639 3644
www.aooa.com.au

Provides information about the olive oil market.

Australian Olive Association
Tel: 0061 8 8535 7170
www.australianolives.com.au

Provides information about olive oil, sets quality standards, and encourages a successful olive industry.

United Kingdom
The Olive Oil Store
Tel: 0044 20 7288 1249
www.oliveoilstore.co.uk

Supplies organic and natural products, including olives and olive oil.

The Olive Store
Tel: 0044 166 1886755
www.theolivestore.co.uk

Supplies olives and olive oil from Andalucia in Spain.

A l'Olivier
www.alolivier.co.uk

Supplies olive oils and related products.

Index